Working Therapeutically with Women
in Secure Mental Health Settings

Forensic Focus Series

This series, edited by Gwen Adshead, takes the field of Forensic Psychotherapy as its focal point, offering a forum for the presentation of theoretical and clinical issues. It embraces such influential neighbouring disciplines as language, law, literature, criminology, ethics and philosophy, as well as psychiatry and psychology, its established progenitors. Gwen Adshead is Consultant Forensic Psychotherapist and Lecturer in Forensic Psychotherapy at Broadmoor Hospital.

Forensic Focus 27

Working Therapeutically with Women in Secure Mental Health Settings

Edited by Nikki Jeffcote and Tessa Watson

Foreword by Jenni Murray

Jessica Kingsley Publishers
London and New York

Extract on p.153 from *Engraved with a Knife* by Wendy Cranmer, Copyright © Wendy Cranmer 2003. Reprinted by permission of the author.

All rights reserved. No part of this publication may be reproduced in any material form (including photocopying or storing it in any medium by electronic means and whether or not transiently or incidentally to some other use of this publication) without the written permission of the copyright owner except in accordance with the provisions of the Copyright, Designs and Patents Act 1988 or under the terms of a licence issued by the Copyright Licensing Agency Ltd, 90 Tottenham Court Road, London, England W1P 9HE. Applications for the copyright owner's written permission to reproduce any part of this publication should be addressed to the publisher.
Warning: The doing of an unauthorised act in relation to a copyright work may result in both a civil claim for damages and criminal prosecution.

The right of the contributors to be identified as authors of this work has been asserted by them in accordance with the Copyright, Designs and Patents Act 1988.

First published in the United Kingdom in 2004
by Jessica Kingsley Publishers Ltd
116 Pentonville Road
London N1 9JB, England
and
29 West 35th Street, 10th fl.
New York, NY 10001-2299, USA
www.jkp.com

Copyright © Jessica Kingsley Publishers 2004
Foreword Copyright © Jenni Murray 2004

RC451.4
.P68
W67
2004

Library of Congress Cataloging in Publication Data

Working therapeutically with women in secure mental health settings /
edited by Nikki Jeffcote and Tessa Watson ; foreword by Jenni Murray.
  p. cm. — (Forensic focus ; 27)
Includes bibliographical references and index.
  ISBN 1-84310-218-8
  1. Women prisoners—Mental health services. 2. Women prisoners—Mental health. 3. Mentally ill offenders—Mental health services. 4. Female offenders—Mental health services. 5. Forensicpsychiatric nursing. I. Jeffcote, Nikki, 1959- II. Watson, Tessa, 1967- III. Series.
  RC451.4.P68W67 2004
  365'.66—dc22
                                                      2003026947

1843102188

British Library Cataloguing in Publication Data
A CIP catalogue record for this book is available from the British Library

ISBN 1 84310 218 8

Printed and Bound in Great Britain by
Athenaeum Press, Gateshead, Tyne and Wear

Contents

Acknowledgements

We would like to thank Gwen Adshead for her support and guidance during the editing process, and Jackie Short and Miranda Barber for their thoughtful review of the manuscript. We want to express our appreciation of all the authors, who have generously shared their experience and knowledge in their chapters. We also thank those we approached who were unable to contribute but who all greeted the project with support and enthusiasm.

Many people have been influential in helping us to develop our understanding of the issues addressed in this book, through academic, professional and personal support. Tessa would particularly like to thank Peter Hutchison, the Watson family (especially Jenny Watson) and the group.

Nikki would particularly like to thank Paddy Bazeley, Stephen Frosh, Sharon Leicht, Leah Murray and Les Petrie for their rich and varied contributions to her thinking about women's needs. The value and good fortune of a secure start in life is a theme that runs implicitly throughout this book; my love and thanks to Tom and Fay Gorsuch for this great advantage. And a special thank you to Peter Jeffcote for his patience, support and good humour, and for making things possible.

Foreword

We all know it's not always easy as women to live up to what's expected of us in the 21st century. We're supposed to run the family, the home and a job and still we struggle with inequalities in the way women are treated, particularly around those everyday issues such as balancing home and family life, or women's lack of equal pay. It's hardly surprising that the incidence of stress and depression is rising. But we rarely encounter women who are experiencing the severe and enduring conditions of mental illness and distress that are described here.

Social changes do not affect men and women equally, and attitudes and responses to disturbed behaviour may vary considerably according to a person's gender and social background. The rhetoric of community care and social inclusion is paralleled by a massive and continuing rise in the prison population and a disproportionate increase in the number of women in prison.

But there are encouraging first steps. There is growing recognition of the lack of expertise and established research concerning women's experiences of secure mental health settings. This is the type of knowledge that is vital if we are to understand more about how services must change if they are to meet women's needs. Indeed, only recently the Government recognised, in its strategy document *Women's Mental Health: Into the Mainstream, Strategic Development of Mental Health Care for Women* (Department of Health 2002a), that women's needs are poorly met because they are the minority in a system mainly designed to support men. Because of this, *Working Therapeutically with Women in Secure Mental Health Settings*, which describes important and innovative work with women who cross the divide between hospital and prison, is timely. It makes an important contribution to the debate about the provision of appropriate services and I hope it will be read widely by both policy makers and practitioners, not least by those who seek to co-ordinate services across traditional boundaries in order to deliver what the service users – those individual women – really need.

Reading of women such as Annmarie, Jemima and Jean (see Chapter 7), we hear shockingly familiar stories. These women have suffered damaging abusive experiences in childhood and adulthood. They have lost children, been rejected by their families, suffered extended periods of severe and enduring mental ill-health and have expressed their distress in desperate acts against themselves and others. Yet there is – still – a lack of understanding of how abusive experiences in early life can affect women's use of, and ability to benefit from, mental health services. The same is true of many women prisoners. Fawcett, of which I am President, is currently working in this area through its Commission on women in the criminal justice system. Meanwhile the contributions to this book seek to understand early experience as it relates to mental health, consider new research, and give guidelines to support therapeutic work with these women.

This is just one example, though a graphic one, of how women's lives and experiences are still so different from those of men. And as someone who has never ducked the 'F' word, I was delighted to see that in the book's varied perspectives and case examples, the authors bring clinical and sociological theory and practice together with feminist understanding. It seems to me that this is critical in exploring the way in which the mental health system can enable women to rebuild their lives.

Not everyone who reads this book will agree with the arguments or theories employed by the writers. But all will be engaged by the compelling stories and compassionate thinking about women and their paths out of mental health services. The book is a breath of fresh air: a valuable attempt to learn more about the often hidden needs of a vulnerable group of women, and about the resources and therapeutic relationships they need to rebuild their lives.

Jenni Murray OBE
Broadcaster and journalist
President, Fawcett

Introduction

Tessa Watson and Nikki Jeffcote

This book grew from the experience of running a women's group on a secure women's ward. Those of us who facilitated the group were moved and impressed by it. We found that, as well as giving to the group, we received much back for ourselves. Afterwards, we were drawn to our memories of the group and the women time and again.

After discussing with the women the idea of documenting the group, we began to write a paper about our shared experience. Contrasting pictures of giving and receiving emerged. One picture of caring, strength, wisdom and resourcefulness, another of pain, loss and disability. One picture of what the women wanted and needed, and another of what services were able to offer them. We wondered about these different facets of the women's and professionals' experience, and asked many questions of each other about how mental health services can negotiate giving and taking, to work meaningfully with each individual woman and provide the specialist services that she needs. From our discussions came the realisation that more literature focusing on this developing clinical area was needed, and thus this book was born. The enthusiasm and energy of all our authors for critical enquiry into the needs of women in secure mental health services has made editing it a profoundly satisfying and moving task.

The book, written for professionals of all disciplines and of both genders, explores ways in which the needs of women in secure settings can be thought about and how these needs may be met through integrated multi-disciplinary work.

Currently, there is no comprehensive evidence base for work with women in secure mental health settings. Theory is developing from practice, and it is thus essential to document the work that is being undertaken. To mirror this process, we have divided the book into three sections: 'Theory-building', 'Practice' and 'Service Development'. Throughout these three sections common themes emerge, and we consider these in more detail later in this Introduction.

The 'Theory-building' section offers different perspectives on the needs and situation of women in forensic settings. It includes clinical, sociological and feminist understandings and discussion of recent service provision and current priorities (Chapters 1, 2, 3, 4 and 5). Key environmental and therapeutic issues are considered in the light of recent research and current service delivery, and these chapters address the ways in which women's and men's needs differ. We welcome a contrasting view in Chapter 6 where Gwen Adshead contributes to the debate, arguing that men and women in forensic mental health services are 'more alike than different'.

In the 'Practice' section, writers from a range of different professions share their experiences of working with women in different settings. They use many clinical illustrations of their work, presenting stories and examples that will be familiar to those who work in similar services. The section begins with an account of a model of integrated multi-disciplinary practice (Chapter 7), which describes, through imagined case studies, three women's care by the multi-disciplinary team, considering the challenges and outcomes that might arise. The chapters that follow describe nursing and therapeutic work with women. These discuss the use of psychodynamic and attachment theory frameworks to consider ways of 'thinking under fire' (Chapters 8 and 9) and include the story of two women's groups (Chapters 10 and 11). The authors in this section describe the impact of the women's ways of being on the team, of wordless communication through self-harm, of shame, and of the desperate wish to be found whilst also hiding. They also draw conclusions from their work, continuing the process of clarifying what women need and find therapeutically useful.

The 'Service Development' section explores the knowledge gained by those working in women's services in recent years that can inform the development of new and future services. It seeks to support teams by offering frameworks and guidelines, and to help those new to this work to avoid painfully 'reinventing the wheel'. Chapter 12 charts the development of medium secure services for women over the last decade. Learning to work therapeutically and creatively with the women while managing the intense feelings that are aroused requires robust and specialist training and supervision (Chapter 13). Particular issues concerning the gender of staff in women's services, and the pressures experienced by both male and female workers, are discussed in Chapter 14, with specific consideration of the role of men on women's wards. The book concludes with a chapter describing the development of Women in Secure Hospitals (WISH), the main voice for women who use forensic mental health services, and describes WISH's advocacy model, which facilitates the power and influence of women over their own care.

KEY THEMES

Readers will be aware that this book, and the questions and issues that it addresses, are timely. The Department of Health's recent document *Women's Mental Health: Into the Mainstream, Strategic Development of Mental Health Care for Women* (2002a) highlights a commitment to the development of gender-sensitive mental health services for women. The document states that 'women's needs are poorly met by being the minority in a system of secure care primarily designed for men' (2002a, p.63). This book gives detailed consideration to the issues raised in *Into the Mainstream*, such as relational and physical security, the therapeutic environment, therapeutic input, listening to women, multi-disciplinary work, staffing and training.

Although we have not tried to present a unitary perspective on the needs of women in forensic services, some themes have recurred throughout the book. One concerns the importance of working together. The need for close co-ordination and communication between professionals, teams and agencies, is described in many different ways. From our own experience, we are aware of the frequent possible disruption to close and positive liaison within teams. These problems in negotiating differences and boundaries are reflections of our patients' difficulties in integration, and can prevent us from keeping the needs of each individual woman in mind. The particular challenges for multi-disciplinary teams working with women are considered in Chapters 1, 7, 8, 13 and 14.

Another key theme concerns the need to remain aware of how women arrive in forensic services and how they can be helped to leave them again. This issue is explored in Chapter 2, where the 'uncharted and uncertain territory' of women's pathways through the services is mapped. The authors describe how women 'struggle and manage to survive damage' despite being exposed to the destructive effects of inequality and abuse. They note the difficulty these women have in negotiating an end to their links with secure mental health services, suggesting a 'sense of life at the end of a long chain which can be hauled in at the least sign of a "problem"'.

Part of these women's journey has been their childhood experience. The early abusive experiences of women who find themselves in secure services are highlighted again and again in repeated statistics and stories of awful physical, sexual and emotional abuse that underpin the women's mental illness and disturbed behaviour (Chapters 1, 2, 7, 8, 9 and 15). The authors repeatedly address the question of how, in the face of such deprived, damaged and institutionalised lives, we can respond to give these women the resources that they need to live their lives in more satisfying ways.

We are drawn to work within this community and wish to provide meaningful treatment for the women with whom we work. Thus the writing and the reading of this book addresses questions for us all about our engagement with women in secure mental health settings. It raises issues that may feel challenging and personal; difficult to consider and answer. It may make us aware of our own identification with these women and our own wish to be known and to hide. Perhaps it will make us more aware of our response to the difficult feelings that, naturally and healthily, arise during the course of our work. It holds up a mirror to the ways in which we manage the pain and trauma that our patients bring us. It also offers practical advice and guidelines which we hope will provide a framework for thinking about and responding to these challenges.

We had hoped to be able to include a chapter written by or with women users of secure mental health services. We wanted these women's voices and stories to be heard strongly in this book in their own words. It has not proved possible to do this, due to dilemmas around confidentiality and the endurance of the written word, and the difficulty of negotiating and respecting boundaries. However, Laila Namdarkhan brings the clear voice of WISH, and its knowledge and advocacy of women's views, to this book. She has encouraging and salutary words: 'It is possible to listen and respond to women and to develop a service that is informed by what they have had to tell us.' We share Laila's concern that more women should be empowered to speak of their experiences and to contribute to the development of services in future.

To conclude, we hope that this book will be a source of knowledge, guidance and ideas for those working, or with an interest in working, with women in secure mental health settings. We will be glad indeed if it gives rise to increasing enquiry and research that will influence the scope and efficacy of the services provided.

Part I

Theory-building

If we had a keen vision and feeling of all ordinary human life, it would be like hearing the grass grow and the squirrel's heart beat, and we should die of that roar which lies on the other side of silence. As it is, the quickest of us walk about well wadded with stupidity.

Middlemarch
George Eliot

1

Thinking about the Needs of Women in Secure Settings

Nikki Jeffcote and Ray Travers

INTRODUCTION

Most readers of this book will be aware that work in secure mental health services for women presents particular challenges and demands. This opening chapter offers a commentary on the relevance and potential of a shared and holistic model or framework for addressing these challenges, and on the benefits and difficulties of such an approach. In this way it aims to set the scene for more detailed discussion of the specific issues that are addressed in the rest of the book.

WHY A DIFFERENT APPROACH FOR WOMEN?

In mental health services, the idea of using explicit models to think about and understand patients' difficulties is taken for granted. The main psychiatric and psychological models – medical, cognitive-behavioural, psychoanalytic (or at least psychodynamic) and systemic – are generally accepted and familiar. A model offers a way of understanding a phenomenon. Provided it does not reify and harden to a supposed statement of 'the truth', it can organise experience and observations in a manner that is intelligible to all team members.

Different models tend to be associated with different professions, and a model may have more or less power and currency depending on who is using it and on the social and cultural context of the work. In forensic mental health services the medico-legal framework, within which patients are detained, privileges the medical model and this can be a source of frustration for other professionals at times. But, by and large, forensic mental health teams are able to integrate their different practices and perspectives without undue conflict.

So what is different about working with women? This chapter discusses the need for teams working with women in secure settings to have some shared understanding of how to think about women's difficulties.

THE UTILITY OF MODELS

Before looking in detail at the needs of women in forensic settings, it is worth thinking more generally about the utility of models. They are useful in facilitating communication between team members and in providing coherence to a team's thinking and interventions. A shared language and a shared approach to conceptualising experience, behaviour and relationships can enhance the potential for reflection and thought by both staff and patients. In some settings, particularly specialist services for individuals with personality disorder, such as therapeutic communities and dialectical behaviour therapy (DBT) programmes, a single shared model is central, providing a clear mutual framework for understanding and addressing experiences and behaviour.

On the other hand, adherence to a model can be constraining and limiting. A 'one size fits all' approach does not do justice to patients' unique histories and diverse ways of dealing with the world. In settings that do operate to a single model, the model's integrity is supported by careful selection of the programme's participants and clear rules as to when membership of the programme is forfeited and an individual excluded. This degree of gatekeeping is not an option for services that take patients on the basis of legal as well as clinical judgements. There may also be complex systemic reasons why shared models tend not to be promoted outside specialist services; for example, professional 'protectionism' and a wariness about practice being open to scrutiny.

THE SALIENCE OF RELATIONAL ISSUES

This chapter is based on the authors' experience that the usual 'multiple model' approach to multi-disciplinary practice in forensic mental health services can inhibit a meaningful understanding of the needs of many women patients. The ways in which, and extent to which, women's needs are different from men's is a highly complex issue. However, perhaps the most salient difference, which has become increasingly recognised over the last decade (although not necessarily reflected in the design and operation of services), concerns the social and relational context both of women's intra-psychic distress and difficulty, and of their actions and behaviour in institutions and the community. It is the authors' view that all aspects of work with women in secure settings – assessment, treatment, rehabilitation, habilitation, facilitation, support, validation and empowerment – should be underpinned by respect for women's actual experience as it is lived and expressed by them, and by a framework that seeks to understand it as socially embedded and socially constituted.

Women who find themselves in secure mental health settings are marginalised physically and psychologically from the social and relationship networks to which they used to belong. The very idea of 'belonging', which represents a balance between inclusion, acceptance and recognition of individuality, has in any case often been highly problematic for women who have commonly experienced abuse, deprivation and neglect during their development. As adults, their mental distress and its attendant behaviour alienate them from the community of women. The stigma they bear is mirrored by internal shame that is by its nature actively hidden. Thus there are powerful external and internal pressures towards ostracism and 'disappearance'. At the same time, women have strong social and relational needs that are somewhat different from men's. Women's orientation to others has been theorised in various ways, from biological accounts invoking genetic and maternal instinctual factors to socio-cultural accounts that draw on social learning theory and gender stereotyping, but its validity as a phenomenon is not in doubt (Gilligan 1982). Women in general have better social networks than men. When these are stable and effective, they protect against mental ill-health (notwithstanding a prevailing culture that prizes independence and autonomy). However, where the ability to form and maintain relatively stable and positive relationships is seriously compromised, women may have few other resources to support their mental and behavioural stability and may still seek meaning and validation in relationships with others.

The prevalence of disadvantaged and damaging early experiences among women who end up in secure mental health services has now been well documented (e.g. Stafford 1999). This work emphasises that women who require 'secure care' have been, and in many respects still are, victims as well as perpetrators. The Government's policy document for mental health services for women, *Into the Mainstream* (Department of Health 2002a), summarises many of the reasons why women may be particularly vulnerable to mental ill-health. These include poverty, social isolation and devaluation of the kind of work, including unpaid caring (i.e. relational work), that women tend to do. Experiences of violence and abuse, both in childhood and adulthood, are more common for women than men and are associated with increased risk of mental illness. Child sexual abuse of girls is more common than of boys, and more likely to be intra-familial. These are all social experiences that impact on social connectedness, sense of self and the way of relating to others.

IMPLICATIONS OF THE RELATIONAL CONTEXT

Staff new to secure women's services are often unprepared for the difference of these wards from the predominantly male wards on which they trained or have previously worked. The highly charged and behaviourally disturbed nature of women's wards can be emotionally disabling to staff. It may be helpful to describe some of the experiences staff are faced with, as these highlight the centrality of relationships and attachments. An inability to think about or address these aspects of the work can contribute to the damaging and at times iatrogenic nature of women's services.

Secure women's services usually have a 'reputation' within their wider organisational setting as highly stressful and demanding places to work. Working with women is recognised as 'different' and staff may therefore also be seen as 'different' and become somewhat marginalised. Specialising in work with women is often seen as a professional cul-de-sac and as indicating a rather suspect 'fluffiness'. Women's wards are known for their emotionally intense atmospheres, very frequent assaults and repeated acts of self-harm that painfully challenge professionals' wish to help and support. Nursing staff often comment that they would rather deal with a physically violent male patient than with the more subtle, complex and covert forms of aggression presented by women. Staff experience intense interpersonal demands. Women patients often approach and engage with staff as soon as they enter the ward, and personal questions are common. Women notice the kinds of relationships staff have with each other; warmth, dislike and sexual attraction between colleagues are likely to be noticed by many of the women long before they are obvious to other staff. The women frequently gain quite intimate knowledge of the lives of staff and may actively use this knowledge in a variety of ways. Because disturbance is often 'catching', a nurse may be assaulted one moment, involved in restraining the perpetrator the next, and attending to another patient who has just self-harmed a few minutes later. Although assaults by women tend to be less severe than assaults by men, they often have a peculiarly personal quality and strong emotional impact. And positive change is often very slow, with many setbacks. Some patients may suddenly and repeatedly lose all the progress they have made – a process that is often termed 'sabotage' and that can create intense feelings of hopelessness, betrayal, bitter disappointment and anger in staff. For other women, nothing seems to change and hope gradually dissipates.

Faced with highly disturbed behaviour, forensic mental health teams typically default to medical approaches, but teams working with women generally find the medical model lacking. The majority of women do not fit easily into diagnostic categories and many have had a range of diagnoses over their psychiatric careers, usually involving some combination of schizophrenia, schizo-affective disorder, mood disorders and personality disorders. This complexity means that a great deal of clinical time and attention can be taken up with debate about diagnosis, in which there is no real increase in understanding of the woman's behaviour and experience. Attempts by individual professionals to introduce different perspectives may only confuse the picture further, and the spaces between different models and approaches can easily become fault lines or fissures dividing staff within teams. The dichotomous nature of medical concepts can be taken up in the service of defensive processes that operate in conditions of high emotional demand. Discussions about the phenomena that cause most confusion and anxiety in teams – violence towards self and others, atypical psychotic experiences and chronic or unusual somatic symptoms – often consist of disagreements as to whether they are 'put on', involving moral and value judgements about women's motivation and character. The complexity of these phenomena, their conscious and unconscious motivations and their intra-psychic and interpersonal functions often disappear from view.

A RELATIONAL VIEW

It is the authors' view that an awareness of relationships – internalised and 'real world' attachment relationships, and relationships within and between systems – is essential to work with women in secure settings. This understanding is needed not only to inform appropriate and helpful therapeutic care to women with complex difficulties, but also to help staff survive the emotional demands of the work and gain satisfaction and meaning from it.

In low secure and general mental health services, neo-Rogerian principles of respect, positive regard and acceptance may often be sufficient. For many women in forensic services this stance may be not only unhelpful but actively damaging. Warmth and acceptance will be meaningless to many women whose very existence as separate human beings has been denied for much of their lives. Staff need a more sophisticated way to think about their relationships with the women if they are to ground themselves and offer therapeutic containment. 'Common sense' assumptions about how people normally or preferably behave towards each other may be irrelevant to women whose hold on reality is fragile and fluctuating and whose life experience has not been consistent with these 'normal' assumptions. Failure to recognise this can lead to women's behaviour being inappropriately attributed to deliberate wilfulness. It can also cause staff to respond unhelpfully and, over time, to become disillusioned.

AN ATTACHMENT-AWARE PERSPECTIVE

Attachment theory (Bowlby 1951) offers a useful set of ideas with which to think about these issues. It has at its heart the idea that human beings are inherently relationship-seeking, and that the primary biological function of attachments is to achieve safety by maintaining proximity to a caregiver. Attachment theory proposes that a sense of inner security is developed interpersonally, through the experience and internalisation of protective and responsive caregiving. It also makes a fundamental link between anxiety and expressions of aggression as a way to regulate relationships. Human babies and small children will die if they are not attended to; being left alone instinctively creates anxiety and arousal, which is expressed in powerful communications of distress, fear and protest to bring back a protecting caregiver. When all goes well, a child learns to modulate and control these instinctive responses. The experience of protection and safety is internalised and children learn to use language as well as action to express and represent their needs, emotions and relationships. Protective attachment figures no longer need to be physically present all the time because they are 'there' in the child's – and later the adult's – mind, where they have a comforting presence in situations of stress.

However, when a child's caregivers do not respond to her anxiety, or respond with rejection, anger or fear, or abuse her physically or sexually, she must find ways of surviving and achieving some sort of safety as best she can. This may mean shutting overwhelming or unacceptable experiences and feelings out of consciousness; heightening her own attachment behaviour to obtain some attention, even if it is punitive or aggressive attention; and becoming highly sensitive to cues given off by others, to help her adapt her own behaviour to their moods and intentions. Where abuse and deprivation have been severe, as they have for many women in forensic services, inconsistency, secrecy and the gap between appearance and reality may significantly impair the ability to know what is real and what is not real. Where there is constitutional vulnerability, this may manifest in adolescence and adulthood in psychotic symptoms that partly incorporate past sensory and psychological experiences that cannot be put into words. The idea of any continuity in others' behaviour may be lacking altogether, or 'caring' relationships may only be understood as exploitative and abusive. Punitive behaviour by others, which at least seems to acknowledge a woman's existence, may represent love to her. Absence of help in understanding her own feelings and responses, and denial or invalidation of those responses, may leave her without any cognitive purchase on her emotions and perceptions. Adverse physical environments, both pre- and post-natally, may reduce the constitutional resources available to her in trying to organise and survive this confusion and chaos.

Empirical studies have in recent years suggested that the consequences of early abuse and deprivation include neurodevelopmental impairment that underpins at least some of these psychological effects. Severe stress in childhood has been shown in particular to disrupt development of the hippocampus and amygdala, which are involved in the formation, retrieval and emotional content of memories. Impairment in the development of these brain structures has been linked with disconnections in consciousness, increased sensory and reduced verbal representation of distressing memories, emotional irritability, and increased anxiety and aggression (van der Kolk *et al.* 1996). The attachment system is partly mediated by endogenous opiates, and high levels of stress in childhood have been shown to reduce the number of opioid receptors in the brain. It has been suggested that this means high levels of stress in adulthood – experienced, for example, in situations of violence (as victim or perpetrator), self-harm and re-enacted trauma – are required for the release of internal opiates and a feeling of internal comfort and relief. Where there are few other available sources of self-soothing, this process may become addictive. These neurophysiological consequences of early abuse may also link to the very high levels of substance misuse and eating disorders among forensic women patients.

A key principle arising from attachment theory and the work associated with it is that behaviour that challenges staff – violence, self-harm, bullying, competition with other patients, smearing excrement, sexual disinhibition – is likely to be functional for the woman in a range of ways: as a means of emotional self-regulation, to experience a sense of agency, to regulate relationships and relationship-distance, and as a communication. Staff often experience strong pressure to conform to the women's expectations of relationships. They will inevitably at times also experience strong anxiety in the face of powerful disturbance, distress and hostility, and may react with overt or covert aggression in their own attempt at self-protection.

IMPLICATIONS FOR PROFESSIONAL PRACTICE

Attachment theory itself is just one model or framework through which some aspects of our work can be thought about and understood. It has been elaborated here because it offers a way of making sense of behaviour and experiences that are easily felt to be overwhelming and incomprehensible. However, no one model will ever be enough and this chapter argues for an attitude, or philosophical stance, that goes beyond any single set of ideas; for a holistic perspective that emphasises connections and links within and between individuals, groups and structures.

If used within this overall attitude or stance, many of the 'mainstream' models have a great deal to offer as staff struggle with both individual and systemic challenges. For example, the therapeutic potential of medication can best be realised if attention is paid to its meaning and context. As well as bringing relief through its psychotropic action, medication is a currency or medium for relationships both with staff (including nurses, who are the main carers, and with high status doctors) and with other women. It may be used to calm staff anxiety and as a substitute for other interventions for which the human resources are not available. It may be used punitively, or may be withheld because a woman's complicated symptomatology does not quite fit the required diagnostic picture. Teams need to have a way of thinking about this level of meaning and process to work most effectively.

Similar contextual and relationship issues apply in the psychological and occupational therapies, which can potentially help women manage, organise and bring structure to some of their needs and experiences. Therapeutic relationships fluctuate and need constant attention, even in the most structured therapies. They will usually involve strong and painful feelings on both sides. Apparent engagement may be misleading, reflecting the woman's expertise at being 'a good girl' and leading the professional into collusion. Lack of engagement can be misconstrued as lack of motivation rather than reflecting a deep sense of worthlessness or fear of being known by another. Relationships with other women and with various professionals will affect a woman's participation at any given time. The therapy itself may at different times, and for different reasons, be seen as desirable, irrelevant or too threatening. Women often experience a strong pressure to 'prove' they always fail.

For individual interventions to be effective, the operation of the whole system around an individual woman, including the continuing influence of her past experiences, her relationships within and outside the hospital and her place in the wider social environment, need to be thought about. Most therapeutic models assume a greater degree of continuity in emotional, cognitive and interpersonal functioning than is the case for many women in forensic settings. Rather than being pathologised, fluctuations in a woman's thinking, mood and behaviour can be taken as opportunities to relate responsively to her and to offer interventions at the right moment.

IMPLICATIONS OF A RELATIONSHIP-AWARE SERVICE

These aspirational ideas must be tempered with realism. Adopting a relationship-aware framework involves considerable challenge and commitment, both for the staff involved and for managers of the service.

First, the approach requires high levels of ongoing support, training and supervision. The pressure to act and react rather than to think and reflect is strong and fairly unrelenting. Proper clinical supervision – regular, consistent and separate from managerial supervision – is needed, both individually and for teams. Finding the resources for this in the face of severe staffing and skill shortages may be impossible. Training at the appropriate level of sophistication and accessibility may also be hard to obtain.

An attachment-aware approach also requires staff to be aware of their own relational styles and of their assumptions about life. We all use implicit models to understand our own and others' behaviour. These models are based on our own particular experience of life and relationships and will reflect our age, family background, culture, ethnicity, sexuality, class and gender. They include ideas about how men and women behave and are different from one another. Because these models will tend to 'take over' in conditions of stress (just as patients revert to their personal, familiar models for understanding the world in times of anxiety and crisis), they are as influential as theoretical and professional practice models. A proportion of staff will struggle with their own difficult histories and with issues of identification and motivation that arise in thinking about women's experience and communications. Providing the structural support and confidentiality necessary for meaningful supervision that addresses such issues is very challenging in restricted environments.

As discussed above, pressures on staff in women's services come not only from patients and from within the staff group but also from the wider organisations within which they sit. Promoting a sense of equality and value in a women's service can be difficult in a society that still pays more, and pays more attention, to men than women, and in organisations where typically the more powerful positions are held by men.

A WORD ABOUT MEN

This chapter has focused on the importance of links, connections and relationships. Making connections involves being alert to resonances between individuals and groups that are generally seen as different. The welcome attention over the last decade to the particular needs of women presents an opportunity to think again about the needs of male forensic patients too.

The great majority of men in secure mental health services, like the great majority of women, have suffered multiply from the effects of social inequalities. They too have frequently had experiences of disrupted attachment relationships, physical, sexual and emotional abuse and failures of care. These experiences may have a different meaning for men, and may differ in their form and consequences, but they are still damaging and we live in a society that remains intolerant of vulnerability in men. It is to be hoped that increased knowledge of the effects of childhood deprivation and trauma, which has received much of its impetus from recognition of the childhood antecedents of borderline personality disorder in women, will be used in a more sophisticated understanding of male as well as female forensic patients.

On a structural and procedural level too, men and women in secure hospitals have many needs in common – a need for treatment choice, for individualised care plans, for meaningful and accessible activities, for information they can understand and for advocacy. Both men and women also require protection and support in relation to bullying and harassment, in whatever forms they occur. The need for safety and the need for respect – which are both, above all, social needs – are part of being human and transcend gender and all other types of difference. They may be achieved in different ways for men and for women, but can stand as common principles in all services. They also link us to all our patients, as they link our patients to us and to each other.

LAST THOUGHTS

Work on attachment shows that fear and anxiety prevent personal development, growth and exploration. In women's services, levels of anxiety are often very high among both staff and patients and there are no easy solutions. We believe that shared attention to the relational context of the work offers the most hope of bringing psychological containment and security to everyone involved. The chapters that follow draw on different perspectives and theoretical backgrounds to explore the range of knowledge, experience, ideas and understanding that may help us towards this end.

2

Dangerous Journeys

Women's Pathways into and through
Secure Mental Health Services

Jennie Williams, Sara Scott and Carole Bressington

INTRODUCTION

Women arriving in secure mental health services, like women entering prison, have mostly lived lives marked by multiple deprivation and abuse. Like prisons, secure mental health services fail to recognise the impact of such lived experience on the thinking, behaviour and emotions of women in their care. The women's pathways are not difficult to map, but to the majority of staff they remain uncharted and uncertain territory. In this chapter we will examine what is known about women's pathways through secure mental health services, using a perspective that directs attention to the effects of social inequalities on women's mental health. This includes the effects of gender, class and race as well as the profound inequality and stigma women experience as patients in secure hospitals. The past, present and future lives of women in secure services are shaped by the intersection of multiple dimensions of oppression.

We begin from the assumption that the abuse and misuse of power matter: that injustice and maltreatment impact on our identities, diminish our confidence, limit our sense of competence and self-efficacy, haunt our memories, and can severely disrupt our ability to live a life fulfilling to ourselves and acceptable to others. We further assume the importance of early relationships and experience in shaping our vulnerability or resilience to later misfortune or maltreatment. There is now a wealth of evidence to suggest that these assumptions have particular significance for women, and hence that it is inappropriate to conceptualise women's mental health problems in terms of individual pathology. It is both more accurate and more useful to conceptualise women's mental health problems as responses to – and sometimes as creative ways of coping with – damaging experiences that are rooted in their lived experiences of inequality and abuses of power (Milne and Williams 2003; Williams 1999).

Social inequalities not only create psychological challenges, but also shape social and institutional responses to the ways that individuals try to manage and survive these challenges. Within the criminal justice system, for example, biases at every stage make it more likely that women will receive a psychiatric disposal than men (Allen 1987; Coid *et al.* 2000). Furthermore, it has been noted for many years that mental health services are no different from other social institutions in having rules and practices that serve the interest of privilege. Hence, services are frequently responsible for compounding the past experiences of disempowerment of many service users rather than providing opportunities for acknowledgement, understanding and change. The central paradox for mental health services is that, at the same time, they are trying to meet the needs of people who are damaged by social injustice (Penfold and Walker 1984). Therefore, it should not be surprising that many mental health workers experience this as very difficult (Parkes 1997; Williams *et al.* 1998; Williams, Scott and Waterhouse 2001), and that there is sufficient dissatisfaction amongst service users to energise an international social movement.

We now examine evidence that will help us understand some of the important ways that social inequalities shape women's pathways through services. This evidence is drawn from research studies, interviews with key informants, and one of the author's (CB) experience both of using secure mental health services and of working with and on behalf of other women travelling this 'dangerous journey'. All three authors also draw upon knowledge gained from providing training to staff working with women in secure mental health services (Scott and Parry-Crooke 2001; Scott and Williams Chapter 13 in this book).

EARLY LIVES

The most revealing information about the early lives of women in the high secure hospitals is provided by Stafford's (1999) study. She carried out a survey and analysis of case register data for all patients resident in the three high secure hospitals in 1997. The findings show that whilst there were exceptions, most of the women were very vulnerable members of largely powerless communities. They came from large working class families: only 16% came from families where the head of household had a professional or white collar occupation. Most had experienced early abandonment or loss of carer followed by problematic attachment to foster/adoptive families resulting in over a third of the women being 'looked after' in children's homes. There was documented evidence of early difficulties in schooling: 23% had been sent to special schools which, as Stafford notes, would have been male-dominated, and 75% had no educational qualifications. Most of the women had only a tenuous grip on the world of employment: over a quarter had never been employed, and 76% were solely dependent on social security payments for their income prior to admission. Evidence suggested that most of these women – over 80% – had not experienced a stable partnership as an adult, so while nearly 40% had children, most were lone parents.

These findings are corroborated and elaborated by other research (Chipchase and Liebling 1996; Dolan and Bland 1996) and also by the case studies prepared by staff as part of the 'Working with Women in Secure Settings' course (see Chapter 13 in this book). As part of this training, staff are required to gather information from records and, when possible, the woman herself about the effects of social inequalities on her life. We have now heard presentations on the lives of over 150 women in secure services. Their early lives are typically characterised by abuse, abandonment, little or no social/family support and financial hardship, followed by a drift into and out of diverse institutional settings where labels of failure are accumulated. Common themes are: violence between parents, alcohol use by parents, transgenerational problems and strong indications of sexual, physical and/or emotional abuse by close family members and others, most of them male. Common early indicators of distress include running away, suicide attempts, alcohol and substance abuse, and being attributed with 'learning disabilities'. Some women make attempts to establish a life for themselves through work though rarely holding down jobs for long periods. A combination of poor education and psychological vulnerability places them at the margins of the workforce where work is typically stressful, unreliable and poorly rewarded. A proportion – 20% in Stafford's study – also form relationships with men. While these relationships often offer women a sense of normality, they are characteristically exploitative and abusive. Those women who have children rarely raise them with the support of a partner, and responsibility for the care of children is usually devolved to other family members or to the state. Some women encounter additional difficulties because they belong to ethnic minorities. In addition to the burden of discrimination, women who have suffered abuse from members of their own community may find it especially difficult to achieve a positive racial identity. Institutional racism also means that most ethnic minority women will find mental health services insensitive or indifferent to their cultural needs. While some women come from economically privileged backgrounds, they have usually endured extreme abuse within highly controlling families; abuse that has been protected from public scrutiny and state intervention by their social status.

Their gender, class and race have taken a great toll on the lives of these women. Initially failed by their families, they have not found support, protection or value anywhere else. They have had very few opportunities to build a life outside their family, and while their distress and behaviour may have been noted, labelled and responded to, their needs have not been met.

What do we know about the ways in which women respond to such levels of abuse, deprivation and abandonment? We know it is inaccurate to use the language of victimology when there is plentiful evidence of their struggle to manage and survive damage that is historical and ongoing. Dissociation, self-harm, eating distress, embodiment, the use of prescribed and non-prescribed drugs, assault and fire-setting, are all common ways that women manage unbearable feelings of anger, anxiety, depression and loss when they have limited control, and when they do not feel entitled to speak or safe enough to do so (Lart *et al.* 1999).

ENTERING SECURE CARE

Many women who have profound experiences of disadvantage and oppression of the kinds that we have just described do not come to the notice of mental health services. This is for a number of reasons. As Warner (2000) observes, many find ways of 'managing their past hurt and successfully negotiate their present adulthood' (p.5). These women are likely to have had access to resources such as money, education, work, and love and support from families and friends: resources which are inequitably distributed in society. Other well documented ways of coping with overwhelming feelings and circumstances include the use of illegal and prescribed drugs, alcohol, and self-harm (Langan and Pelissier 2001). Some of these women will become visible to mental health services, though they may be deflected on grounds of untreatability or 'failure to engage'; others will come to the attention of the criminal justice system (Carlen 1998; Singer *et al.* 1995), or drug and alcohol services. Mental health services are not the only social institution struggling to manage women who are experiencing high levels of psychological distress.

Research shows that people enter mental health services in a range of ways including through choice, coercion and 'muddling through' the difficulties of life (Pescosolido *et al.* 1998). However, we have been unable to find any research that has asked women themselves how they come to 'end up' in secure mental health services. Anecdotal evidence suggests that some women idealise the potential of maximum security to provide them with asylum, safety and sources of expertise. However, we rely here on studies that have looked for evidence from case register data, records and questionnaires from staff. What can we learn from them?

With few exceptions most women enter *maximum* security health provision from other institutions: in order of frequency, from prisons, medium secure units and NHS hospitals (Coid *et al.* 2000). Women transferred from prison have been charged with, or convicted of, an offence. Admission without a conviction from other mental health services is typically mediated by difficulties in managing the woman's behaviour in that setting, including violence to staff, fire-setting and self-injury, in that order.

Women enter *medium* secure health provision from, in order of frequency, prison, NHS hospitals, the community, and high secure hospitals (Coid *et al.* 2000). Where there is no conviction, the behavioural difficulties precipitating admission involve violence, self-injury, absconding and fire-setting, in that order.

Most women who enter secure services are, as Lloyd (1995) observed, 'doubly deviant, doubly damned' for contravening expectations of their gender as well as the rules of acceptable social behaviour. It is their behaviour that determines the women's entry into secure services, which respond with regulation, security and medication. This behaviour can also be read as evidence that these women have not had their mental health needs met by mainstream mental health services. They have not been provided with the safe, therapeutic relationships – the relational security – that would enable them to begin talking about their unspeakable experiences, experiences which have usually included further traumatisation in an array of 'care' services. Transfer to secure services gives women perimeter security which it is widely acknowledged few need (Department of Health 2002a); they need relational security which could, and should, have been provided much earlier in their pathway through services.

MOVING AROUND SERVICES

It is probably the exception rather than the rule for women to get their needs met by mental health services (Williams, LeFrancois and Copperman 2001). This is hardly surprising when diagnosis hides the connections between a woman's behaviour and distress and her lived experience. Without an understanding of these connections, behaviour is easily viewed as meaningless, out of control and dangerous. Yet we cannot hope to empower women unless we have an understanding of their disempowerment.

As we have noted elsewhere (Williams, Scott and Waterhouse 2001) there are common threads in the ways in which mental health workers in community and secure services account for their lack of response to the needs of women service users, in particular their reluctance to provide women with safe opportunities to talk about their histories of trauma and deprivation. First, many report that they have not received the kind of training that would enable them to respond in this way and do not have access to appropriate supervision and support. Second, many staff believe that the competence, opportunity and responsibility for providing therapeutic help to women with histories of trauma and deprivation lie elsewhere in the service system. However, while there are dedicated staff working within mainstream mental health services who have made it their business to develop the skills to provide effective help to women (e.g. Gorsuch 1999; Watson, Scott and Ragalsky 1996), they are far fewer than service providers would like to imagine. These prevailing beliefs often result in women being passed from service to service, some through increasing levels of security where their distress often escalates.

That emotions and behaviour originating in profound experiences of disempowerment increase on admission to secure settings is unsurprising (Chipchase and Liebling 1996; Heney and Kristiansen 1997; Lart et al. 1999). These are settings in which anxiety, anger, guilt and feelings of powerlessness are likely to increase rather than decrease (Milligan, Waller and Andrews 2002). For some women this is exacerbated by lack of contact with their children and concerns about their competence as mothers (Houck and Loper 2002). Coid et al. (2000), following their comparative study of men and women, comment on the manifest changes in the behaviour of women admitted to secure care. However, these authors' commitment to the concept of 'personality disorder' invites us to conclude that this could be something to do with women's pathology rather than an understandable response to their environment: 'Many personality-disordered women have an observed tendency to manifest more disturbed behaviour in secure settings, including deliberate self-harm, and where the presentation of their clinical symptoms can be exacerbated' (Coid et al. 2000, p.292).

Psychiatric labels supplemented with ward-based jargon are the raw material of women's reputations. This information, together with details of their index offence, precedes them into all settings. Labels also obscure a woman's needs, add to her day-to-day derogation and massively reduce staff creativity and optimism (Perkins and Repper 1998). We find huge consistency throughout secure services in the language used to talk about women and their difficulties. One of the tasks on the 'Working with Women in Secure Settings' course is to generate these terms; having done so, participants often comment that it is difficult not to feel disempowered and rejecting when a woman is described in these ways at handover or in a referral form. The huge effect that this can have on women patients is neatly summed up by one of the women speaking in a recently launched video about women and mental health services: 'For a long time being described as a hopeless case had an intensely depressing effect on me' (Mental Health Media 2002).

Participants on the 'Working with Women in Secure Settings' course are also asked to think of alternative ways of speaking that are respectful and informed by an understanding of women's disempowerment. Some responses to this exercise are listed in Table 2.1. These responses suggest that change in secure mental health services could be achieved if, and when, staff are trained and supported in the development of an honest appreciation of the histories and backgrounds of the women with whom they work. Such a change would need to be underpinned by increased sensitivity to the implications of the great disparity of power between staff and service users, and a real commitment to making this work in the interests of women patients.

Table 2.1 Better Ways of Speaking

Jargon and labels	Better ways of speaking
Attention-seeking	She is trying to build relationships
Borderline personality disorder	She is doing her best despite early experiences of deprivation and trauma
Controlling	She doesn't always want to do what staff want her to do
Dangerous	She *sometimes* behaves in ways that put herself and/or others at risk
Devious	She doesn't feel able to ask for what she wants directly
Hormonal	There is a remote possibility that she sometimes experiences difficulties associated with hormonal changes
Immature	She seems young for her age
Malingering	She is 'somatising' her distress
Manipulative	She doesn't believe that she is entitled to get her needs met if she is open about what she wants
Masochistic	She expects to be hurt by others and sometimes finds it easier to provoke a response than to wait for what she believes inevitable
Paranoid	She experiences the world as very threatening and can feel very unsafe
Personality-disordered	She is emotionally distressed, has low tolerance of frustration, and relies on coping strategies developed in situations of great deprivation
Secretive	She protects her privacy
Suspicious	She is not at the point of trusting us yet
Unco-operative	She doesn't like doing what staff want her to
Untreatable	We are finding it difficult to help her.

LEAVING SECURE CARE

The literature on the process and consequences of leaving secure care is almost non-existent, reflecting a widely-shared lack of interest in women's lives after discharge. For example, the current development of single sex secure facilities for women is rarely accompanied by investment in 'step down' facilities. It is widely recognised (Lart *et al.* 1999) that even when women are assessed as needing a lower level of security, they frequently have to wait for long periods of time, sometimes years, before a place becomes available. This is particularly likely to be the case for women who have an index offence relating to arson, even though the overwhelming majority will not have intended to endanger life or destroy property (Stafford 1999). Nonetheless, within care settings and secure services, the risks are viewed seriously.

Changes in the woman's behaviour are a requirement for transfer to a less secure setting. This is commonly described by both staff and the women themselves as 'going through hoops'. Some women find the resources within themselves to do this, and find support from staff and the other women with whom they live. They may well have experienced care and advocacy from some staff, and the importance of this should not be under-estimated. However, few women will have received psychotherapy (Chipchase and Liebling 1996), and so will not have been enabled to talk about their lives in ways known to be healing (Harris 1998; Scott 2001). We therefore have a situation where women have passed through the entire system, which for most represents many years of their lives, before being allowed to leave with all of their presenting problems intact. One of the authors (CB) went to Broadmoor and emerged much the same woman; essentially nothing had changed except the growth of her own self-garnered survival skills.

At present, few women or men living in high secure accommodation are discharged into the community on either an absolute or a conditional discharge. Stafford's (1999) survey found that the majority of women were transferred from high security to other psychiatric hospitals. Transfer is rarely needs-led and arrangements could generally be described as ad hoc. Transfer is dependent on what placements and funding are or are not available. Differences in availability can make the experience feel like a lottery.

The preparation for transfer offered to women also varies with each setting and staff group. In some instances staff are very committed and careful in addressing the practical and psychological considerations of transfer. They can be very robust in challenging a woman's reputation and supporting her right to a better life. A few services provide sensible practical courses of rehabilitation skills, but even when women are 'ready' for transfer they may find themselves waiting months or years to move on. In other cases, the preparation offered to the women is negligible and staff expectations are low; in such instances women are prepared and briefed for 'failure'. This is commonly associated with an 'out of our hands now' approach, and a lack of interest and advocacy for the future of the women. Women have been told: 'We'll keep your bed for you, you'll be back.'

Women who go to secure units that are predominately occupied by men may have particular difficulties that sometimes lead to failure of the placement. There are many accounts of women who have been sexually assaulted and raped, and then returned to a more secure environment where they have waited for years for another opportunity to be transferred. They tend to be blamed for these events and it is often seen as their failure. It is at such a point of heightened levels of fear and distress that some women choose suicide as an alternative to going back through the process again. The message – that it is dangerous or too difficult out there – is very demoralising for the women and for staff who shared their hopes and aspirations.

One of the most serious problems for women following transfer to lower levels of security is the history they bring with them, or which often precedes them: histories which are usually suffused with high levels of stigma. Often the very worst is assumed of them by people who know and understand the least; a fusion of discrimination and ignorance that follows them all their lives. Information about their index offence and/or behaviour is widely shared. Mezey and Bartlett (1996) suggest that women who have been civil patients and have no index offence may be particularly vulnerable in this respect, as unchallenged descriptions of behaviour are placed on their records.

Women who leave high secure hospitals can be very eloquent about the demands of transition from this level of security and the consequences of living for long periods of time, sometimes many years, in a high secure environment. The day-to-day practices relating to, for example, physical security, locking doors, mixing with staff and other patients have become a way of life. Many women do not feel prepared for transfer and do not understand what is required of them; there is a great deal of fear and anxiety about 'What am I meant to do?' For example, one of the authors (CB) remembers standing by a canteen door, being unable to open it and walk through, but feeling 'too stupid' to explain why. Many staff at secondary placements are not aware of, or do not want to acknowledge, the depth of institutionalisation arising from living for long periods of time in a high secure environment. Few realise the extent of de-humanisation of life in a high secure institution. Women have led lives that have been rigorously policed. Privacy is not something they get as a right; it has to be earned, and every part of their lives is open to scrutiny. Their mail is censored, their clothes are chosen for them. All the basic, everyday domestic minutiae are left behind when they leave high security and the huge impact of this is rarely acknowledged in ways that women find enabling. This is especially important in the early days following discharge when a woman's capacity to manage and make choices in her new environment comes under close scrutiny.

The process of discharge can be described as an obstacle course. However, it is usually seen as risky and dangerous for those who are operating the system, not for the woman. Staff expect her to fail and look for evidence that she was not ready to transfer, that she cannot cope, or that she is in the wrong place. They often feel the same as did the staff involved in the women's original transfer to high security – that they are not able to deal with these kinds of problems and should not be expected to. These beliefs can co-exist with an accepted wisdom that such women cannot change and that they are somehow taking valuable resources away from 'genuinely mentally ill' people who might otherwise benefit.

Very little is known about those women whose pathways from secure provision lead to the community, other than information that has been gathered by WISH (Women in Secure Hospitals). This group of women is hard to track. This may be because, once they are free of statutory restraints, they put as much distance between themselves and mental health services as possible, which is not nearly as difficult as it sounds. Many rarely, if ever, access services again and are assumed to have made a successful transition back into the community simply because they have disappeared. Available evidence suggests that community services are very reluctant to offer help or assume responsibility for women in this position. Many years after leaving

Broadmoor, one of the authors (CB) moved to a part of London where she coincidentally knew someone working in mental health services. He later said that had he known then about her 'history' he would have 'run it up the local services flagpole' on the grounds that 'they needed to know there was someone like her living in the borough'. Little wonder, then, that many women go to extraordinary lengths to conceal their history. The damage thus wrought in women's lives reverberates into the next generation, and into relationships of every kind. The history might be concealed but it cannot be forgotten and women know the risk of exposure. Many keep it secret from friends, colleagues, even their partners and children, which places them under a constant burden of anxiety and guilt. A fundamental factor in the lives of post-secure women is the very deep and rational fear of being sent back, and they experience a sense of life at the end of a long chain which can be hauled in at the least sign of a 'problem'. So what for most of us might be a bad patch or an event occasioning stress, becomes for these women a high risk situation requiring particularly resourceful self-management.

WISH has responded to an obvious gap in service provision by setting up a community project, which is London-based in the first instance. This Department of Health-funded project offers practical help and advocacy to women who are about to leave, or are at risk of entering, secure provision. Women refer themselves to the project, or are referred by others; some will have got to know WISH through the services they provide in the secure system.

CONCLUSION

Within the context of secure services, women are seen as risky and dangerous and are endlessly scrutinised and judged with this in mind. Instead, as we have shown, the dangers are located in the woman's past and present experiences of profound disempowerment. These women will never fit neatly into diagnostic systems, and have little hope of progressing their lives in pharmaceutically-reliant service contexts. They are still being victimised by Victorian systems and approaches to containment, and by paternalistic regimes that ignore and hide the significance of social inequalities. An honest recognition of the dangers of women's pathways through secure services represents an important starting point in closing the gap between women's needs and the responses of services. Encouraging signs that this is beginning to take place can be found, for example, in the mental health strategy for women (Department of Health 2002a) and in the conclusion of the following review of women and secure services:

> Women's civil and human rights are violated in a number of ways: the level of security at which women are held, inappropriate treatment, delays in transfers and discharge, as well as issues relating to privacy, dignity, security and protection from harassment and sexual or physical assault. (Lart *et al.* 1999, p.7)

Ignorance – in the face of the evidence reviewed here – no longer serves as an excuse for the failure to take action. As long as mental health services generally, and secure services specifically, continue to ignore the effects of social inequalities and place reliance on individual pathology and diagnosis, women's pathways through these services will continue to be often unnecessary, dangerous and too long.

3

Women and Offending

Helen Rutherford

INTRODUCTION

Women commit a relatively small proportion of all crime and represent a minority of those held in prison. The relationship between women's offending and mental disorder has been the subject of uneasy and unresolved debate at least since the 1970s, when an attempt to reorganise and rebuild HMP Holloway as a secure hospital failed (Maden 1995).

A number of studies over the last decade have looked in detail at mental disorder in prison and have identified a high level of unmet need among both women and men. However, over the same period the overall prison population has risen substantially, with a disproportionate increase in the number of women. This chapter aims to review women's offending, the current situation of women in prison and the possibilities for more appropriate provision for female offenders.

WOMEN'S OFFENDING

Women commit less crime than men, their offences are less serious and committed less often and women's criminal careers are shorter (Heidensohn 1996). Of women born in 1953 in England and Wales, only 8% had a conviction before the age of 40, compared with 34% of men, and 1% had received a custodial sentence, compared with 7% of men. More women have only one conviction. Figures for 2001 reveal that cautions or convictions for acquisitive offences accounted for 60% of female offending, as against 36% for men; for violence the figures were 9% and 12% respectively and for drug offences 10% and 20%. Among the female sentenced prison population, the main offence groups were drugs (39%), acquisitive offences/fraud (20%), violence (15%), robbery (8%) and burglary (5%) (Home Office 2002a).

THE INCREASE IN THE PRISON POPULATION

Following an unprecedented rise in prison numbers over the last decade, the UK now has the highest rate of imprisonment in Western Europe. In the 11 years to November 2002, the total prison population in England and Wales rose by 63% to nearly 73,000. Over the same period, the number of women prisoners rose by 180% to a total of 4,364, representing 6% of the prison population (Home Office 2002b).

These higher rates of incarceration have not been matched by increased rates of offending; the total number of both male and female offenders found guilty or cautioned for indictable offences fell between 1992 and 2001, the number of women falling by 13.4%. Women committed fewer offences of burglary, theft, handling stolen goods and violence against the person, but more robbery, fraud and forgery, and criminal damage. Drug offences increased by over 50%. While the total number of women dealt with by the courts has increased over this period, the proportion dealt with by the Crown Courts has remained fairly stable. The escalation in the female prison population is therefore not the result of an increase in serious offending; rather, it is due to changes in sentencing policy. A Home Office report suggests that the rise in sentenced prison receptions for women 'is being driven by a *more severe* response to *less serious* (sic) offences' (Home Office 2002a, p.21).

New legislation that has driven up prison numbers includes the Criminal Justice Act 1993, which advocated greater use of immediate custody for indictable offences and increased sentence length at both Magistrates' and Crown Courts, and the 1994 Criminal Justice and Public Order Act, which introduced tougher sentences for young offenders. These changes have affected both men and women and reasons for their disproportionate effect on women are unclear. A contributory factor may be the over-use of remand to prison (pre-trial and pre-sentence) for women by Magistrates' and Crown Courts. Fewer female than male remands ultimately receive custodial sentences (29% in 1994, compared with 44% of men, but increasing to 41% and 50% respectively in 2001). The shortage of bail hostels for those with no fixed address has been cited as an element of this problem (e.g. Cavadino and Dignan 1997), and may be more acute for women who require gender-appropriate, safe accommodation.

As noted above, recent data indicate that the increase in sentenced female prison receptions has been driven largely by a greater readiness to impose custodial sentences for less serious offences. Custody rates for female offenders sentenced by the Crown Courts have nearly doubled in the last ten years, while women sentenced in Magistrates' Courts were subject to custody *five times* as often in 2001 compared with 1992 (Home Office 2002a). This may be due partly to a lack of practice guidelines within the Probation Service for ensuring that women have equal access to community sentences. However, Hough's (2003) analysis of sentencing trends confirms the increased use of imprisonment where a community penalty would previously have been given. Guidelines to magistrates in the Halliday Report (Home Office 2001a) recommended that prison sentences be extended to less serious crimes; as offences such as theft and handling, fraud and forgery are more often committed by women, these guidelines may therefore have contributed significantly to the disproportionate rise in the numbers of women in prison (Hudson 2002).

In 2001, sentence length for three-quarters of female offenders was between three months and one year. As well as many more women serving short sentences, prison numbers reflect longer sentences for other women, particularly for drug offences. Sentencers are also reluctant to impose fines on women, resulting in an increase in the use of community penalties, which render women vulnerable to imprisonment at an earlier stage (Worrall 2000).

THE CRIMINAL JUSTICE SYSTEM AND ATTITUDES TO WOMEN'S OFFENDING

Notwithstanding these increases in the use of custody, the evidence for differential attitudes towards men and women within the criminal justice system portrays a complex picture.

It has often been suggested that women are treated more leniently than men. In the 1980s, Allen (1987) showed that women received more sympathetic and individualised justice for serious crimes than men. Carlen (1983) found that women conforming to conventional roles, for example, those married with children, were treated more leniently by the courts than single mothers, who were considered to have transgressed gender norms.

A more recent review of sentencing concludes that most women are treated more leniently than male offenders, with the exception of first-time violent offenders and recidivist drug offenders, who are treated equally (Hedderman and Gelsthorpe 1997). This study found that magistrates distinguished between 'troubled' and 'troublesome' offenders, tending to view women as 'troubled'; usually first-time offenders facing less serious charges who behaved more respectfully in court. For this group, measures such as discharge or probation predominated.

Home Office statistics reveal that women are less likely than men to be remanded into custody or committed for trial, although this is to some extent accounted for by differences in offence type and history. Following arrest, women are more likely than men to be cautioned and less likely either to have no further action taken or to be charged. Over half of female offenders dealt with for indictable offences were cautioned, compared with about a third of men. Women were more likely than men to be discharged or given a community sentence for indictable offences and less likely to be fined or sentenced to custody (Home Office 2002a). These findings suggest that women are indeed treated differently from men by the criminal justice system, but that characterising their treatment as either harsher or more lenient is overly simplistic.

As discussed further below, one consistent area of difference between male and female prisoners relates to the greater use of psychiatric disposals for women, with proportionately more women than men being transferred from prison to hospital. The greater readiness to see women's offending as linked to mental disturbance is also reflected in the use of psychiatric defences (e.g. diminished responsibility) in the case of women who kill

(Peay 1997). Courts are reluctant to accept that a woman may act out of self-defence or as a result of provocation, preferring to find an abnormal mental state ('temporary insanity') in women who kill partners who have battered or abused them. 'Cumulative provocation' is only gradually becoming accepted as a defence for women who kill their partners after prolonged periods of abuse (Hudson 2002).

SOCIAL DISADVANTAGE AND ETHNICITY

Gender is only one dimension of difference reflected in the criminal justice system and other differential characteristics may affect women differently from men. All prisoners are more likely than the general population to have grown up in care, to come from a disadvantaged family and to have experienced poverty (Social Exclusion Unit 2002). However, in terms of educational disadvantage, female prisoners are more likely than their male counterparts to have no qualifications (61% compared with 49%) and to have been unemployed in the 12 months before custody (71% compared with 50%). Over a third of the women interviewed by Her Majesty's Inspectorate of Prisons for England and Wales (1997) had experienced educational difficulties and 20% had spent time in care. A majority lived in rented/council accommodation and subsisted on state benefits, augmented by criminal activity or casual work.

Black people are over-represented in the prison population, which is partly explained by the high levels of social exclusion they experience (Social Exclusion Unit 2002). At end-June 2001, black prisoners comprised 21% of the female prison population compared with 13% of the male prison population. Of black and ethnic minority women prisoners, 19% were foreign nationals compared with 10% of men. Many foreign nationals are women convicted of drug importation, who are sentenced to long periods of imprisonment and suffer significant isolation from their families.

WOMEN IN PRISON

The female prison estate

At the time of writing, 19 prisons hold women. Two of these, Buckley Hall and Downview, previously held men, and three are shared with men. One maximum security (Category A) prison, Durham, has a female wing. Seven prisons hold women on remand (pre-trial/pre-sentence). Three prisons – Askham Grange, Drake Hall and East Sutton Park – hold women in open conditions. Three women's prisons hold girls aged between 15 and 17 (termed 'juveniles') and seven hold young female offenders aged between 18 and 21. To accommodate rising numbers, two further women's prisons, both private, are planned at Ashford, Middlesex and Peterborough, which will together provide an additional 810 places.

HMP Holloway has the largest operational capacity of the women's prison estate, at 492 places. The annual cost per prisoner ranges from £14,376 at Drake Hall to £37,595 at Holloway.

Discipline within women's prisons

During the 1990s, prison regimes became more restrictive following riots and breakouts from male prisons (Cavadino and Dignan 1997). Security and control were increased, leading to tougher regimes. These measures were applied equally to the female prison estate, regardless of women's lesser security needs.

Women have higher rates of disciplinary offences recorded against them compared with men (Maden 1995; Home Office 2002a). It has been suggested that regimes operate a lower threshold for rule-breaking by women, displaying a greater tolerance for men's infringement of the rules (Carlen 1983). Prisoners who breach prison rules are assessed by prison medical staff as to whether they are 'fit for adjudication', that is, mentally and physically able to appear in front of a governor for their case to be heard. For those found guilty, punishment includes loss of association (socialising with other prisoners when cells are unlocked). More harshly, the prisoner may be subject to a period of detention in solitary confinement on the segregation wing. Additional hardships can be imposed, such as the removal of mattresses from cells during the day, and more severe sanctions include transfer to another prison. In the past, prisoners could lose remission, with days or weeks added to the sentence, but this procedure has been discontinued since the European Court of Human Rights ruled that it violates the individual's right to a fair trial as prisoners have no legal representation at adjudication (Ezeh and Connors v. the United Kingdom).

Women with mental disorder who breach prison rules are not usually segregated in solitary confinement, due to their mental illness and risk of suicide. They are usually made 'unfit' for adjudication and their cases dismissed. Exceptionally, women with mental disorder whose behaviour proves unmanageable may be held in segregation, occasionally for lengthy periods of time. Despite daily review by prison medical and nursing staff, these women's care falls below an appropriate standard and reflects the difficulties achieving hospital transfer for certain groups, for example, women with severe personality disorder.

Special groups within prison

Young women

UK legislation has increasingly provided for the imprisonment of children, through the Criminal Justice and Public Order Act 1994, Crime and Disorder Act 1998 and Criminal Justice and Police Act 2001. This situation has prompted the United Nations Committee on the Rights of the Child (UNCRC) to express concern over the escalation in rates of child imprisonment in the UK (Goldson 2003).

A review by Her Majesty's Inspectorate of Prisons (2001) found that sentenced girls were being held in units for 18–21-year-olds and that unsentenced girls were accommodated with adult women, a breach of the UNCRC. The girls spoke of bullying and criminal contamination due to their location on adult wings. The Inspectorate raised concern over lengthy confinement in cells and the availability of drugs. It subsequently criticised the failure of HMP Holloway to provide adequate regimes and appropriate physical environments for girls, with little awareness of child protection procedures and no assessments of vulnerability (Her Majesty's Inspectorate of Prisons 2003). The Youth Justice Board has stated that all 15–16-year-olds are to be placed in non-prison service accommodation during 2003, although 17-year-olds will continue to be held in prison (Atkinson 2003).

Mothers in prison

Lack of contact with their children is one of women prisoners' greatest concerns. The Inspectorate's (1997) review of women in prison found that two-thirds were mothers; that over a third had one or more children aged under 5 years and 55% had at least one child under 18 years. Four women's prisons – Holloway, Styal, Askham Grange and New Hall (which houses juveniles) – currently provide mother and baby units, with a combined capacity of 80, and a further 46 places are planned. Argument continues over the age at which babies should be separated from their mothers in order to prevent institutionalisation by exposure to the restricted prison environment, and 18 months is currently seen as the limit. The Home Office has no current plans to develop units for women with older children. The Inspectorate's recommendation for overnight visits by children to mothers in prison has not been implemented, due to lack of appropriate accommodation (Home Office 2001b).

Mentally disordered women

A study by Maden, Swinton and Gunn (1994) of the sentenced female prison population showed higher rates of mental disorder among women than men. Although the prevalence of psychosis was similar, at a little under 2%, women had higher rates of personality disorder, substance misuse and learning disability. A later study by Singleton et al. (1998) found a prevalence rate for psychosis of 14% among all female prisoners, compared with 7% for male remands and 10% for male sentenced prisoners. Fifty per cent of women met criteria for a diagnosis of personality disorder compared with 78% of male remands and 64% of male sentenced prisoners. The different findings of these two studies may be due partly to their different populations and different methods of assessment, but may also reflect some real increases in morbidity due both to social changes and to the adverse effects of overcrowding as prison numbers have grown. Most studies have found borderline and antisocial personality disorders to be the most common among women prisoners.

Studies have consistently found higher rates of substance misuse among female prisoners compared with men. Singleton et al. (1998) reported dependence on drugs in 41% of female sentenced and 54% of female remand prisoners. The Inspectorate's report on HMP Holloway (2001) found that 45% of new female receptions were in need of immediate detoxification and that 50% seriously abused alcohol.

As already noted, one consistent area of difference between men and women in prison relates to the higher rate of transfer to hospital for women. However, the actual number of women transferred is very low compared with the estimated levels of psychiatric morbidity. Despite the Home Office policy that mentally disordered offenders should receive care and treatment from health and social services rather than custodial care, increasing numbers fail to achieve transfer to psychiatric services (Reed 1992; Maden 1997; Reed 2003). A study in HMP Holloway carried out in 1995 (Rutherford and Taylor in press) showed that less than 2% of remand prisoners were transferred to hospital. Women who had committed the least serious offences and who transferred to open psychiatric wards, spent up to five weeks in prison. Women with a diagnosis of personality disorder spent three times longer in prison than women with mental illness before they were transferred to hospital. Factors accounting for this included the more serious nature of their offences and difficulties finding beds.

It has been suggested that the higher rate of transfer of women than men to hospital may not so much reflect the meeting of women prisoners' mental health needs as reflect a more punitive attitude to male prisoners.

Studies by Dell *et al.* (1993) and Gorsuch (1998) shed some light on the reasons why women referred by prison psychiatrists to NHS services did not always obtain beds. Both studies found that most women with a clear psychotic illness obtained beds, while women with prominent personality difficulties or a learning disability had most difficulty obtaining placements. In Gorsuch's study, 'difficult to place' mentally disordered women were characterised by chronic self-harm and sexual abuse in childhood and commonly had extremely deprived and abusive backgrounds, as well as lengthy criminal histories. Among those women who failed to obtain a bed in both studies, arguments about treatability, the degree of security required and the necessary length of treatment were common. A number of authors have noted that psychiatric reports may be selective, allowing forensic mental health services to reject patients they do not want (e.g. Maden 1997; Reed 2003). Some of the women rejected by the NHS and given custodial sentences prove to be among the most difficult to manage within the prison estate.

Arson is more common among female than male offenders with mental disorder. Explanations for this include the suggestion that arson allows the expression of anger without physical confrontation. Women who committed arson in Gorsuch's (1998) study had diagnoses of personality disorder, histories of sexual and/or physical abuse and were difficult to place in NHS psychiatric facilities. Women admitted to secure forensic mental health services under the legal category of 'psychopathic disorder' are more likely than those detained under 'mental illness' to have been charged with arson (Coid *et al.* 2000).

It has been noted since the 1980s that women may be remanded to prison as a route to treatment for their psychological and social difficulties (Edwards 1984). There is some evidence that the practice of inappropriate remand to prison for medical or psychiatric reports continues (Prison Reform Trust 2003). Dell *et al.* (1993) concluded that it was 'useless, as well as inhumane' (p.643) to remand women for this purpose, and this observation appears to be as true ten years later.

Self-harm and suicide in prison

Self-harm is common among female prisoners and ranges from minor self-inflicted scratches, excoriation with scourers, overdose or swallowing objects to life-threatening cutting or self-strangulation.

Prisons have historically used 'strip' cells for self-harming or suicidal women; this involves seclusion in single cells furnished with a mattress and cardboard furniture and the use of strip dresses (long garments of heavy, overstitched fabric secured by Velcro) to prevent further acts of self-harm. This response has been recognised as punitive and anti-therapeutic and other measures recommended, such as the use of shared accommodation and provision of psychological help to facilitate greater understanding of self-harm and the development of coping strategies.

Risk factors for suicide include previous self-harm, substance misuse and mental disorder, all of which are common in prison populations. Suicide is increased in remand prisoners and those recently sentenced (Leibling 1992), and occurs at quiet times during the day and night, when prisoners are locked up (Shaw, Appleby and Baker 2003). Despite the provision of specific training to staff, suicide rates among women prisoners are rising at an alarming rate. Nine women killed themselves in prison in 2002 and during the first six months of 2003, ten women have committed suicide (Prison Reform Trust 2003).

Impact of prison on women

Imprisonment of women has a disproportionate impact on family stability and ties, and causes considerable anxiety and distress to the women themselves. The separation of children from mothers in custody is now recognised as a cause of inherited disadvantage (Home Office 2001b). Research has established that serious and persistent young offenders are more likely than other young people to have weak family links and to have spent less time with their parents (Social Exclusion Unit 2002). The social costs of women's imprisonment are therefore as high as (and compound) the financial costs.

The brevity of many women's prison sentences allows little rehabilitative work to be carried out. Recent research indicates that prison does not prevent recidivism (51% of women and 58% of men are re-convicted within two years) and that short sentence length (less than 12 months) predicts higher re-conviction rates (Social Exclusion Unit 2002). Women find it hard to obtain employment after release from custody and 'Pathfinder' projects, which act as a bridge between custody and the community, have been developed for short-term female prisoners to facilitate their search for work after release.

Prison regimes readily re-invoke past trauma for those who have been victims of abuse. This is reflected in the high levels of disturbance and self-harm in women's prisons, which create considerable stress both for prisoners and for officers who are not trained to manage severe mental disorder and its behavioural concomitants. Awareness training programmes for prison staff working with women with histories of abuse are not widespread.

THE GOVERNMENT'S STRATEGY FOR WOMEN OFFENDERS

The Government's Strategy for Women Offenders consultation document (Home Office 2001b) recognises that factors such as poor health, economic instability, lack of employment and training opportunities and experience of abuse are criminogenic for women. Curiously, the negative impact of imprisonment on children is acknowledged, whereas the impact of prison on women themselves is overlooked. Risk is central to the Strategy, which has the stated aim of protecting the public and reducing re-offending. Custody is to be reserved for women who 'really do need to be there'. Through the Women's Offending Reduction Programme (WORP), the Government aims to improve offenders' access to work, tackle drug use and improve family ties and the life chances of young women. The Strategy sees lack of cognitive skills as central to women's offending; however, the emphasis on cognitive skills programmes has been criticised (Hannah-Moffat and Shaw 2000) and recent evidence suggests these courses may be ineffective in reducing recidivism (Hough 2003).

CONCLUSIONS

The Government's reliance on imprisonment as punishment has been criticised as harsh and ineffective. Critics have proposed the use of alternative penal systems, for example, based on the principles of restorative justice, which places victims at its centre and reduces the use of imprisonment to a minimum.

Prison remains an unnecessary and excessive punishment for most women. The range of community penalties available, including home detention curfews (HDCs), which allow short-term prisoners to complete their sentences at home, and drug treatment and training orders (DTTOs), should reduce the need to imprison women, although, predictably, the demand for places in drug detoxification units exceeds supply, resulting in custodial remands.

As noted above, there is still little NHS provision for women prisoners with personality disorder, and their prospect of receiving any sustained programme of treatment within prison is limited. Current Home Office initiatives include a pilot of dialectical behaviour therapy (DBT) in a small number of women's prisons and a therapeutic community for women at HMP Winchester. There are considered to be too few women who meet the criteria for 'dangerous and severe personality disorder' (DSPD) within prison and high secure hospitals to justify a dedicated service (see Chapter 5 in this book). Women offenders with severe personality disorders will continue to receive lengthy custodial sentences.

Many women resent the stigma attached to a psychiatric disposal, preferring to serve a prison sentence. There is an urgent need to develop an appropriate female remand facility and to support the therapeutic community at HMP Winchester. More generally, early intervention and accessible and appropriate mental healthcare is needed in prisons. Expansion of court diversion schemes would expedite admission to hospital for offenders who are acutely ill and/or at risk of suicide, but the principal reason for difficulties in transfer from prison remains the shortage of secure psychiatric beds (Reed 2003).

Ultimately, restricting the use of imprisonment to those offenders who pose a risk to the public would reduce prison numbers and allow the Prison Service to meet the recommendation of the Joint Prison Service and NHS Executive Working Group that prisoners should have access to healthcare of an equivalent standard to that available to the general population.

4

Troubled Inside:
Vulnerability in Prison

Jackie Short and Miranda Barber

She had been made to break an accepted social law, but no law known
to the environment in which she fancied herself such an anomaly.

Tess of the D'Urbervilles
Thomas Hardy

INTRODUCTION

As discussed by Helen Rutherford in the previous chapter, there are more
women in prison than ever before, and the number is rising. The popularity
of TV dramas such as *Bad Girls* suggests a growing interest, and perhaps a
perverse fascination, with women in prison. To those who work in the real
world, it is clear that the criminal justice system lacks the appropriate
resources to address the problem of women's offending. Prison is a
male-dominated environment, run primarily for men by men, with levels of
procedural and physical security that are less relevant for women's containment. Breaches of security frequently result in a blanket tightening of
security measures across male and female prisons, with a disproportionate
impact on female prisoners. Research into offending and 'what works' has

drawn predominantly upon data from male offenders, and most facilities and programmes have been designed with men in mind.

Women's offending needs to be understood in the context of the roles that women play in society, and to which they may return. Many women in prison have been victims of crime. Whilst it is simplistic, and wrong, to view female offenders purely as victims, it is equally unwise not to recognise and work with the prevalence, in women's histories, of exploitation, significant loss, and poverty. It is also essential to acknowledge the enormous social cost of women's offending and imprisonment in terms of the disruption of family and social bonds.

It is acknowledged that women's experiences of social exclusion and deprivation are intimately linked both to offending and to mental health problems (Department of Health 2002a). It is therefore not surprising that there are a significant number of women in prison with disabling mental health difficulties. However, healthcare in prison continues to fail both male and female mentally disordered offenders. Women bring with them into the prison system chaotic life experiences and mental health vulnerabilities, with high rates of depression, mood disorders and traumatic stress. Substance misuse is a particular problem; many women enter prison self-medicating with illicit substances in an attempt to deal with high levels of stress and poor mental health. For many vulnerable women, certain aspects of prison life, such as loss of privacy and seclusion, add to a sense of loss of control and further exacerbate their difficulties.

Despite the high level of psychiatric morbidity, screening procedures on reception to prison often fail to detect serious mental illness, particularly in those with major psychoses without accompanying behavioural distur-bance. Established medication regimes may become disrupted, causing a deterioration in mental state that often goes unnoticed on the wings. These problems are often compounded by difficulty in obtaining clinical informa-tion from health agencies outside prison, and the lack of a centralised record keeping system within the prison system itself.

TOXIC ATTACHMENTS AND TRAUMA RE-ENACTMENT

Women whose repeated experiences of separation, trauma and loss have made them vulnerable may experience imprisonment as a shock to the system. The prison environment recreates feelings of disempowerment and separates women from those to whom they may be significantly attached. Faced with these experiences, women may use a range of survival strategies. These include avoidant behaviours such as dissociation, self-harm and substance misuse, and extremely chaotic behaviour that fluctuates between intense demands for attention and closeness and abusive rejection and attack. Some may disintegrate into psychic turmoil and psychosis.

Attachment (Bowlby 1951) is the propensity to make strong affectional bonds to others. Women do not, in the main, seek separation, but attempt to build up a sense of connection with others. When separated from family, friends and partners, those lacking strong affectional bonds may form toxic attachments to other inmates and prison staff. The need to belong can be met by forming bullying gangs, or through collective involvement in self-harm and substance misuse.

Prison staff may find themselves becoming favoured by some women and rejected by others, often leading to splits in staff teams and inconsistent responses to women's needs. Staff often have limited training in the mental health needs of female offenders, and little awareness of the presence, or impact, of these toxic attachment patterns. The women's behaviour may be interpreted as 'manipulative' and evoke dismissive or punitive responses in staff.

To reduce offending behaviour, women need help to develop a more secure sense of self, and of self-worth, through the experience of being valued by others. This can be difficult to achieve, however, in a custodial system designed to contain and punish.

VULNERABLE GROUPS

Women are not a homogeneous group, and are individually affected by imprisonment in different ways. There are, however, certain groups for whom the experience of imprisonment may be particularly traumatic. We focus here on the particular vulnerabilities of adolescents, pregnant women and mothers, older women and women who are foreign nationals.

Adolescent girls

There is much concern about the plight of adolescent girls who are housed with adult female prisoners. It used to be argued that housing girls under the age of 18 with adult female offenders was in their best interests, as the older women would 'mother' them. However, the inappropriateness of mixing adolescents with adult females in the prison environment has been increasingly recognised. Many adolescent offenders have already experienced profound deprivation and trauma and an adult prison environment can further damage them. Teenage experience is critical in the formation of gender and sexual role identity, and in the development of a sense of self. It is developmentally appropriate for adolescents to want to test out boundaries and power dynamics; however, such behaviour in adolescent offenders is often not tolerated by either staff, or other older inmates. An example of this is the case of a 16-year-old girl who was beaten up by two adult women prisoners for insisting on playing her music too loudly. Whilst older female inmates may be capable of mothering, the distinction between this and subtle forms of bullying and exploitation can be difficult to make. In addition, the impact of a criminogenic environment cannot be underestimated.

Adolescent prisoners' sense of isolation is often compounded by being placed long distances from their home, making it difficult for family and friends to maintain ties. These difficulties may be complicated by the adverse effect of the girl's criminal behaviour on parents and friends, who can find themselves ostracised by the local community. Adolescent offenders may already have complex and conflictual relationships with family members and relationship partners. In some cases, family members or friends may be the victims of the crime. This presents particular challenges for the girls' reintegration and rehabilitation.

As noted by Rutherford (Chapter 3, this book), the Government has made a commitment to removing girls from the prison establishment, and to placing young women under the age of 21 in Young Offender Units. However, there have been delays in implementing these policies and a significant number of adolescent offenders are still incarcerated in adult establishments.

Pregnant women and mothers

Being pregnant in prison is fraught with difficulty. Accommodation is often not appropriate to the needs of an expectant mother and the prison regime makes little allowance for pregnancy. Ante-natal provision can be a lottery, with some women able to access facilities and care outside prison while others are reliant on ante-natal support being provided within prison. Partners may be excluded from attending routine scans due to concerns about security. There are also well-publicised cases of women being handcuffed while receiving ante-natal care, causing embarrassment and distress both to the woman and to those who are treating her.

While still placed in the main part of the prison, pregnant women may be vulnerable to physical and emotional attack from other inmates, as their condition may evoke strong feelings and unresolved issues in others.

Pregnant women may be faced with loss of responsibility over the future of their unborn child. Women who offend are frequently viewed as unfit mothers, and imprisonment often results in their losing custody of their children, either temporarily or permanently. Attendance at childcare case conferences and possible civil proceedings is restricted and the mother often has little opportunity, in reality, to influence outcomes. For those women who wish, and are able to keep their baby in custody, there are insufficient mother and baby places. Even if a woman is fortunate enough to secure such a place, she faces traumatic separation when her baby is either nine or 18 months of age. Women who have experienced abuse and deprivation, and whose children are placed in care, or with potentially abusive family members, may suffer acute distress and fear that the cycle of abuse will be played out again.

Women with young children outside prison face a number of pressures. Even in emotionally secure families, relationships are disrupted by imprisonment. Women may be placed at long distances from their children and may be moved between prison establishments without notification to their families. Youngsters who do visit have to face both long journeys and seeing their mother in a confined environment. The procedural security of prison, for example, the experience of being searched, can be alienating and frightening for children. The experience of repeated separations may adversely affect the development of a secure attachment to the mother, particularly if the child is young. It is recognised that children with these experiences may develop problematic peer relationships, and are more likely themselves to become involved in the criminal justice system (Baunach 1985). However, there are examples of good practice where prisons offer extended day visits, which give mothers an opportunity to engage in day-to-day parenting activities and may mitigate the damaging effect of separation.

For the mothers themselves, the loss of a central role in their children's lives can be unbearable and may increase the risk of self-harm and suicidal behaviour. This distress is often most acutely expressed at key dates such as children's birthdays, Mother's Day and Christmas.

When release is imminent, successful family reintegration depends on mothers having somewhere safe and secure to live, with enough money to support themselves and, perhaps, their children. However, imprisonment leaves some women with even more damaged attachments to their families and home community, and others may be homeless. For these women, negotiating the challenges of securing appropriate housing and financial resources, while attempting to resume parenting responsibilities, can be very difficult. For mothers returning to families which have adjusted to life without them, reintegration can be painful. Unless provided with support, these women may again face many of the problems which in the past led to behaviours such as substance misuse and offending, and they may quickly relapse.

Older women

Although the number of older women in prison is small, the increasing rate of female imprisonment, and lengthier sentences, means that the age of the female prison population is gradually increasing. This causes difficulties for older women, who may find themselves further marginalised in a regime designed primarily for young men. Wahidin (2000) found that overcrowding and limited resources led to the needs of younger women being prioritised in terms of access to education and opportunities in prison. This left older women with immense difficulties in finding employment upon release. With reduced work opportunities in prison, older women struggled to finance items such as phone cards which would enable them to keep contact with the outside world and preserve their attachments. Older women may face reduced contact with children after they have reached the age of 16, and may lose the opportunity to develop relationships with grandchildren. They may have to cope with the death of parents. Their partners may also succumb to ill-health and relationships may not withstand the stress of separation. Older women who entered prison from a network of family bonds may face the prospect of being alone upon release.

Increasing age brings the menopause, marking the end of childbearing, which may be extremely distressing for women without children. Despite the greater risk of physical ill-health, particularly cancers of the breast and cervix, older women may not have access to appropriate screening facilities in prison. They are often unable to purchase dietary supplements to gain protection against the risk of osteoporosis. Hypertension may go unde-tected, as may the onset of depression, dementia, or paranoid psychosis. Psychological distress may be exacerbated by sensory and cognitive impair-ment. Yorston (1999) notes the difficulty in moving elderly mentally disor-dered offenders to appropriate healthcare facilities, as regional secure units and locked psychiatric wards are generally not designed to meet the needs of older patients.

Foreign nationals

Women who are foreign nationals most commonly find their way into prison in the UK for drug smuggling, being exploited to act as 'mules' for organised drug criminals. Many have come from countries where women struggle to survive against economic and social oppression. Heaven (2000) notes that many are single mothers, in dire financial circumstances. They describe being coerced or deceived into carrying illicit drugs by landlords or moneylenders. Many travel with no money and inadequate clothing, and in custody there can be difficulties and delays in obtaining basic clothing such as underwear.

In her review of the needs of foreign nationals in UK prisons, Heaven (2000) highlights the failure of prison staff to recognise or acknowledge cultural needs, such as dietary requirements and practices necessary for religious observance. The women may have little or no command of English, and are further disorientated by a culture that is alien to them. They may be exposed to racist abuse from prison staff and other inmates, and be unable to communicate their distress. They can have difficulty accessing facilities in prison, such as sport, education and healthcare. Maintaining contact with families overseas is often problematic, due to the high cost of telephone calls. For some, telephone communication is not available.

Women who are foreign nationals have often experienced considerable psychological trauma prior to arrival in this country and are potentially more vulnerable to depression, traumatic stress disorders and major psychoses. Language problems and a lack of interpreters exacerbate the risk of mental illness remaining undetected. Even when they have completed their sentence, many foreign nationals find themselves subject to lengthy immigration procedures, often remaining in prison for several months while they await deportation.

An example of positive practice is Hibiscus, a charity jointly funded by the Prison Service and private trusts, which provides support and material assistance to foreign nationals and their dependants. Overall, however, resources are limited and it can be difficult to raise and maintain cultural awareness in relation to women who are foreign nationals or from minority ethnic backgrounds and cultures.

THOUGHTS FOR THE FUTURE

The criminal justice system struggles to meet the needs of those women for whom it is responsible. Providing effective offending programmes and comprehensive services to address their complex difficulties remains problematic. Periods of custody can have a negative impact on women's lives, result in a deterioration of mental health and increase interpersonal and economic difficulties. While women's offending cannot go unsanctioned, more needs to be done to address the rising numbers of women entering prison.

Alternatives to custody for women who commit less serious crimes could include gender-specific, community-based programmes linked to probation, and the use of supervised group housing. For those whose crimes require detention in custody, the time spent in prison should be kept to a minimum, with additional periods of supervision in the community. Changes in the provision of prison healthcare are already underway with the creation of joint NHS/Prison Service-funded multi-disciplinary 'inreach' health teams, which aim to work in partnership to improve mental health services to prisoners. At present a number of women's prisons have inreach teams, but more needs to be done to implement the substantial programme of change that is required.

Training to raise awareness of the needs of women prisoners, particularly those who are vulnerable, should become an integral part of prison staff induction and continuing professional development programmes. In addition, specialist training and support is required for those working with the most acutely disturbed and disturbing women, some of whom have been rejected by mental health services as 'untreatable'. This would involve enabling and supporting staff to respond appropriately and consistently to the women's challenging behaviour, so that they do not unwittingly recreate potentially collusive or abusive relationship patterns. Containing and transforming toxic attachments is not easy in any setting, and this is particularly the case in prisons, where the institution's primary task is to impose physical security rather than provide emotional security.

Women's offending is everyone's business; it impacts on families, communities and society as a whole and represents one way in which disadvantage is transmitted across generations. Statutory providers of education, health, housing and social services need to work in partnership with criminal justice and voluntary agencies to address the personal, social and economic circumstances that lead women to offend. Within prison, greater attention needs to be given to the groups of vulnerable women discussed in this chapter, to support them through their time in custody and enable them to reintegrate into their communities.

5

Women and Risk

Tony Maden

INTRODUCTION

Women in secure mental health settings present a range of risks to themselves and others, both on the unit and after discharge or release. Measurement of these risks is an inescapable part of care. We need ways of knowing when, and under what conditions, it is possible to relax supervision or to advise discharge from detention. This process is risk management. As it is unavoidable, the only question is how well it can be done.

Risk assessment evolved from the concept of 'dangerousness', by way of risk prediction and assessment. The old approach was to identify dangerous or high-risk patients, who would often be detained for long periods of time with little attempt to define precisely the risks involved. We now recognise that risk has many dimensions. Assessment aims to define risk in terms of the outcome we are worried about, for example, violence, arson or self-harm. The next step would be to define the risk more closely. What type of violence? Can likely victims, or classes of victims be identified? (One of the main gender differences is that women's violence is less likely to be directed at strangers.) Risk assessment shades into risk management, as we go on to consider the factors that may increase or decrease the risks, or to identify early warning signs.

Clinical services have always been involved in risk assessment, but the process has become more explicit and, in many services, more formalised. Where there was once reliance on clinical 'feel' or impression, there is now likely to be a structured or standardised scale. Still, whatever the approach, our concern is with future behaviour, and one theme of this chapter is that accurate prediction is impossible. The best that we can hope for is to identify and manage risk factors, with the intention of ensuring the best possible outcome for the patient. Another theme of the chapter will be the extent to which standardised assessments can help us to achieve this goal. For the most part, I concentrate on risk to others. Similar principles could be applied to any risk, but the standardised assessment of risk to self is less well-developed and researched.

WHAT IS STANDARDISED RISK ASSESSMENT?

Mental health services in the UK were slow to take up the formal assessment of risk but they are now making up for lost time. Both managers and clinicians have embraced the technology of standardised risk assessment, as an alternative to reliance on clinical impressions alone. This is a welcome development, as clinical judgment depends so much on the individual skill and experience of the clinician and is often unreliable. Standardised methods also offer the possibility of objective assessments, free from bias arising from gender, ethnic or class differences between clinician and patient.

Even so, a general welcome for these structured methods should not blind us to their limitations. The first problem is that it is not possible to draw conclusions about an individual from the behaviour of populations. The second problem, of most relevance here, is that there may be problems in applying standardised risk assessments to women.

Dealing briefly with the first issue, standardised risk assessments are based on the behaviour of populations. Individuals do not reliably behave according to expectations. In other walks of life, the principles of standardised risk assessment would be rejected as gross stereotyping. For example, crime rates in many societies vary with ethnic origin. Most people condemn as racist the drawing of conclusions about the criminal tendencies of an individual from her or his membership of an ethnic group, and we need to bear in mind similar reservations about actuarial risk assessment. It is for this reason that the ideal practice is generally considered to be structured clinical judgment. Actuarial or standardised data inform the clinical assessment, but they should not be allowed to constrain or dominate it.

These reservations apply to all risk assessment but there are particular problems when assessing risk in women. The first problem is that standardisation, in risk assessment, usually means standardisation on men.

DE-MYSTIFYING STANDARDISED RISK ASSESSMENT

There has been a rapid proliferation of risk assessment instruments which can be bewildering for the newcomer to the area, faced with a vast range of unfamiliar acronyms. This mystification of the subject is unhelpful. In fact, the variables associated with offending can be reduced to a few underlying themes.

Leaving aside male gender, which has the strongest statistical association with offending, the most important guides to risk are previous offending, childhood behavioural problems, personality or personality disorder, substance misuse, and mental state. Personality disorder is very important. The MacArthur study of ordinary psychiatric patients found that psychopathy, as measured by the Psychopathy Checklist Screening Version (PCL:SV), was the best single predictor of violence (Monahan et al. 1999). Most standardised assessments are variations on these themes, offering greater or lesser emphasis to particular features or ways of measuring the underlying construct.

The important point is that if one has done a thorough clinical assessment of these factors (including a detailed reading of past records) then a standardised measure is not going to introduce much, if any, new information. It may help with the organisation of the information, and it will allow an easy comparison with a reference population. There is also an argument that if one has already collected this information as part of a detailed clinical assessment, it will not take long to fill in a standardised assessment, so one may as well do it. However, this is a convincing argument only if one can be reasonably confident that the particular instrument is a valid measure of risk in women, as I discuss in more detail below.

For many services, it may be that the main benefit of introducing standardised assessment is that it necessitates a full review of the historical and clinical information available on a woman. In the same way, there are indirect benefits of learning standardised risk assessments. One may not always choose to use the specific measure, but knowledge of what is necessary shapes one's clinical practice, and encourages routine collection of the necessary data.

STANDARDISATION OF RISK ASSESSMENT INSTRUMENTS

The principles of standardisation are simple enough, even if the statistics can get complicated. One gives the test to a large group (the larger the better), one waits to see who offends or re-offends, and one attempts to link scores on the test to re-offending. The difficult, and expensive, practical problem is to give the test to enough people to ensure meaningful results. It is impossible to determine the differences between offenders and non-offenders if one has very few offences to study. This leads to an immediate problem in attempting to standardise these tests on women. If violent offending is 20 times more common in men – a conservative estimate of the true difference – then the sample of women would need to be 20 times larger in order to get the same number of offences. As this implies a similar increase in time and costs, it is not surprising that most of the work has been done on men.

The problem is more than the fact that the work has not yet been done, in which case the solution would be to get on and do it. Because rates of some types of offending are so low in women, it may never be possible to obtain large enough samples. The obvious examples would be serious violence against strangers and sexual offending. These offences are so rare in women that standardisation of a risk prediction instrument could never be done to the same level as in men.

APPLYING EXISTING INSTRUMENTS TO WOMEN

How much do these problems matter to the clinician? In practice, they force us to rely on instruments that have been standardised mainly on men. Some are more likely than others to give reasonable results when applied to women, as discussed below. In all cases, we need to be aware that the degree of uncertainty associated with a standardised assessment is higher with women. This means that a full, holistic clinical assessment of a woman must always be used to put the test results in context. As noted above, structured clinical judgement dictates that this same principle is applied when assessing a man, but it becomes even more important with a woman.

Despite the problems outlined above, the good news is that many violence risk assessment instruments seem to do a reasonable job of ordering women in terms of relative risk. In other words, women with higher risk ratings on these instruments tend also to do less well in terms of future violence than women with lower scores. Used in this way, standardised measures may help us to direct our efforts within the clinical team. Given two cases that look similar clinically, we should probably be more cautious in managing the woman who scores highly on a risk instrument, compared to the one with a low score. In this way, the standardised assessment may help us in developing a clinical risk formulation.

Problems arise when an attempt is made to obtain an absolute measure of risk or to compare a woman's scores with men's scores – which is what happens when using norms, if they are based on male populations. For example, it cannot be assumed that a given score on a test means the same for a woman as it would mean for a man. However, this need not be a serious problem, so long as it is recognised. In fact, two men with the same scores may be very different from each other, so the real mistake is to assume that one can conclude too much about any individual on the basis of a single test score.

SPECIFIC RISK ASSESSMENT INSTRUMENTS

Some examples will help to illustrate the issues involved. I have chosen two well established instruments. The Violence Risk Appraisal Guide (VRAG) (Harris *et al.* 1993) claims to predict the risk of violent offending. The Psychopathy Checklist Revised (PCL–R) (Hare 1991) is a measure of psychopathy and not a risk assessment as such, but it correlates highly with risk of violence in many populations. In considering these scales, I am not going to resort to a lot of complicated statistics – partly because the definitive data are not available on women. I shall concentrate instead on face validity. How useful do these scales look, in the light of what we know about offending and risk?

The Violence Risk Appraisal Guide (VRAG)

This is a well researched instrument but an added reason for choosing it as an example is that its authors poked a stick in the clinician's eye by claiming that it is so good at predicting risk that it should not be contaminated in any way by dirty clinical judgements (Quinsey *et al*. 1998, p.171). The following comments can therefore be seen as the clinical retaliation. The VRAG was intended to be a pure measure of risk, untainted by theory or clinical prejudice. It was based on 600 men released from a high security hospital in Canada and followed for seven years. From the masses of information collected on each patient before discharge, which data predicted violent re-offending? The answers – reduced to 12 factors – are shown below:

VRAG factors indicating higher risk:

1. PCL-R score
2. Problems at junior school
3. Personality disorder
4. Alcohol abuse
5. Separated from parents before age 16
6. History of non-violent offending
7. Never married
8. Failure on prior conditional release

VRAG factors indicating lower risk:

9. Age
10. Schizophrenia
11. Extent of victim injury
12. Female victim.

Dealing first with general concerns, even a casual glance at these items suggests that something is not right. We know that psychopathy, conduct disorder and early childhood maladjustment are related to violence risk, so it is no surprise that they feature, but three of the four items indicating reduced risk of violence do not make clinical sense. Older offenders are usually less worrying than younger ones, but should any clinician be reassured because a patient has schizophrenia, caused serious injuries to a previous victim, or chose to attack a woman rather than a man? How did these factors come to be included in the scale? The explanation lies in the nature of patients released from high security hospitals, the group on which the scale was developed. Some are mentally ill, others have personality disorder and, in general, the mentally ill (properly treated) present fewer problems of re-offending. Hence, patients with schizophrenia carried lower risk in this group, but only because they were compared with patients with severe personality disorder. Most literature suggests that schizophrenia increases the risk of violence in both men and women e.g. Swanson *et al.* (1990).

The appearance of victim gender and the extent of injury as violence risk factors in the VRAG also results from the quirky nature of this particular sample. Many of the patients in the VRAG sample had schizophrenia. The victims of offenders with schizophrenia are often close family members, typically mother or spouse. It is likely that this is to do with women having a greater role as carers, and therefore having more face-to-face contact, rather than any specific misogyny on the part of the mentally ill. Whatever the precise motivation, the offence is often driven by strong emotions that are specific to the victim. Removal of the victim in itself decreases the likelihood of re-offending and, combined with effective medication, is associated with a low risk of recidivism.

By contrast, psychopathic offenders who cause serious injury or death to female victims, e.g. violent sexual predators, present a much higher risk of re-offending. But they had little influence on the development of the VRAG because they are much less likely to get out of a high security hospital. They were under-represented in the sample of discharged patients on which the VRAG is based. Therefore the VRAG may convey the misleading message that a female victim indicates a lower general risk of violence.

This speculation is supported by empirical evidence. Many serial killers of women, who have already demonstrated their ability to offend repeatedly, achieve low scores on the VRAG. This is not a trivial problem, as this scale effectively minimises the importance of misogyny as a risk factor for violent recidivism.

More gender-specific problems relate to the application of particular items in the VRAG scale to women. The factor 'failure of conditional release' is less useful in assessing risk in women, because women are much less likely to have had a previous conditional release, so have had no opportunity to fail. Women are also less likely to have a history of non-violent offending. Therefore the presence of either item in a woman may be more significant than in a man, precisely because they are so uncommon. Equally, their absence may carry less reassurance than the same finding in a man. This sounds complicated, but it adds up to less certainty in prediction of future violence in women.

The Psychopathy Checklist – Revised (PCL–R)

The Psychopathy Checklist, later to become the Psychopathy Checklist–Revised (PCL–R) (Hare 1991), resurrected psychopathy as a useful clinical entity by allowing reliable diagnosis. Using this 20 item scale, it was possible to distinguish psychopathy from criminality. And once the condition was defined, it could be researched. There has been exponential growth of research using the PCL–R, well documented on Professor Hare's website (www.hare.org). In summary, scores on the PCL–R have been found to correlate with violence in samples drawn from a range of criminal justice and psychiatric populations and cultural and ethnic groups (Hart 1998).

The PCL–R gives a score from 0–40. Each of its 20 items is scored 0 (absent), 1 (probably or partially present) or 2 (definitely present). A screening version, the PCL:SV, has also been developed, using only 12 items to give a maximum score of 24. Both versions of the scale make use of both case notes and an interview, and can be completed using case notes alone. This gives the PCL an enormous advantage over other measures of personality. No matter how sophisticated, most such measures rely on self-report, a serious problem because lying is a feature of psychopathy. Even if lying is not involved, self-report implies a degree of insight and self-reflection that is beyond the capacity of many patients. The PCL is unique in recognising and measuring the tendency to deceive self and others.

The 20 items that make up the Psychopathy Checklist Revised (PCL–R) are:

1. Glibness/superficial charm
2. Grandiose sense of self-worth
3. Pathological lying
4. Conning/manipulative
5. Lack of remorse or guilt

6. Shallow affect
7. Callous/lack of empathy
8. Failure to accept responsibility for own actions
9. Need for stimulation/proneness to boredom
10. Parasitic lifestyle
11. Poor behavioural controls
12. Early behavioural problems
13. Lack of realistic, long-term goals
14. Impulsivity
15. Irresponsibility
16. Juvenile delinquency
17. Revocation of conditional release
18. Promiscuous sexual behaviour
19. Many short-term marital relationships
20. Criminal versatility.

For present purposes, let us take it for granted that the trained rater can give reliable estimates of the presence of these features. What do they mean? Do they mean the same in women as in men?

It is important to note that there are no gross gender differences in the significance of these factors. Features such as pathological lying, impulsivity or juvenile delinquency are not good signs in women, any more than in men. However, there are more subtle differences, many of which relate to the lower prevalence of offending in women. Factors such as juvenile delinquency, criminal versatility and revocation of conditional release occur less often in women. Also, judgments as to the presence of some characteristics (e.g. promiscuity, irresponsibility, parasitic lifestyle) are bound to be influenced by gender stereotypes.

In summary, then, application of the PCL–R to women may not cause gross errors or distortions but one would have to be aware of a greater uncertainty about the meaning of a particular score. In fact, this is precisely what is emerging from studies of the PCL–R in women. It is useful for ordering or ranking women relative to each other, with higher scores correlating with a greater risk of violence or other offending (Hare, personal communication). There is, however, no basis for assuming that scores are equivalent in women and in men. One cannot assume that a woman who scores 25 presents the same level of risk as a man with a similar score. Once again, the standardised test result needs to be incorporated within a full clinical assessment.

DANGEROUS AND SEVERE PERSONALITY DISORDER (DSPD) AND WOMEN

Recently, the Dangerous Severe Personality Disorder (DSPD) initiative in the UK has revitalised research and service development for men with severe personality disorders who present a risk to others. The picture for women is more complicated, and the benefits of the DSPD programme for them are less clear.

The working definition of DSPD is that an individual must:

1. have a severe disorder of personality

2. present a high (>50%) risk of causing serious physical or psychological harm from which the victim would find it difficult or impossible to recover, and

3. the risk of offending should be functionally linked to the personality disorder.

There is an exclusion clause for serious mental illness, as the services developed under the DSPD initiative are intended to be for severe personality disorder rather than co-morbid syndromes involving psychotic symptoms. It is also stipulated that standardised risk assessment instruments should inform the assessment of risk.

The aim of the service is to protect the public from a relatively small number of dangerous offenders with severe personality disorders, so the threshold is set very high. It is concerned mainly with sexual and violent offending and there are close parallels between this initiative and Violent Sexual Predator (VSP) legislation in the USA. This implies that women are a secondary consideration within this initiative as, even when they are mentally disordered offenders, they have never posed the same level of threat to public safety as men.

It is pointless to go looking for DSPD women using sophisticated risk measures. The criminal statistics tell their own story, with a male:female ratio of the order of 125:1 for sexual offending. The statistics for violence show a lower discrepancy, but it is still high. Even those statistics exaggerate women's threat to public safety, as much of their serious violence is within a domestic context and lacks the predatory element that underlies the DSPD concept.

The conclusion that the number of women meeting DSPD criteria is very small has been reached from first principles, simply by considering the well known facts about women's offending: that they offend at a lower rate than men overall; that their rates of violent and, particularly, sexual offending, are lower still; and that their victims tend to be those with whom they are in a close relationship. This appears to be borne out by Home Office research into likely candidates for a women's DSPD service. It is envisaged that this service will be limited to one specialist prison, and that fewer than 20 women in the whole country will be eligible. Compare this to the DSPD service for men, with a planned 300 high secure beds split between prisons and hospitals and the expectation of long waiting lists, with additional supporting services for DSPD men at lower levels of security.

In one sense, it is reassuring that very few women will get the DSPD label, which has a lot of negative connotations. On the other hand, DSPD is the main development in secure services for personality-disordered offenders, involving a massive resource commitment. The positive side of the development will be a transformation of psychological treatment services for this group of patients, with much greater use of cognitive behavioural programmes. It is not clear that women will derive much benefit from any of this.

This is an unfortunate failing, as the main problems in treating women as mentally disordered offenders are well recognised. I would summarise them as follows:

1. Providing specialist treatment at an appropriate level of security which, for most women, will not be high security.

2. Resolving diagnostic problems, as there is a greater overlap between personality disorder and mental illness than is usually the case in men.

3. Deliberate self-harm co-existing with risk to others, often related to the experience of abuse in the distant or recent past.

None of these problems sits easily within the DSPD framework, which is primarily concerned with public safety. Public safety is not a significant public health issue in relation to women. The danger is that this new initiative will distract attention, and divert resources, from well recognised problems and attempts to solve them. For women who are mentally disordered offenders, DSPD looks like a solution to a non-existent problem.

CONCLUSIONS

The cautious use of standardised assessments of risk can improve clinical formulation for women in secure care but it should be seen as an aid to good clinical practice, not a substitute for it. A good clinical team will be familiar with a range of instruments, and it is unreasonable to expect that any one will prove definitive. It is not possible to use these tools, on their own, to give an accurate prediction of the absolute level of risk in an individual.

6

More Alike than Different

Gender and Forensic Mental Health

Gwen Adshead

We are more alike than we are different.

Jacob Moreno

INTRODUCTION

It is a central contention of this book that female forensic patients need different services from those offered to men. Jeffcote and Travers (Chapter 1, this book) suggest that the contemporary multiple models of care on offer to male patients fail to address the relational needs of women, their marginalisation, and the impact of their experiences of victimisation. These authors argue for different approaches to care for the two sexes.

In this chapter, I wish to put a somewhat different and perhaps unortho-dox view: that male and female forensic patients are more alike than they are different. I want to argue that, although there are real differences between male and female users of mental health services in criminological terms, in other important ways they are similar groups who face similar challenges and difficulties. This is not a general comment about men and women in mental health systems or about men and women in general. Rather, I make a specific claim: that within forensic mental health services, gender does not adequately differentiate between users' needs, and that more sophisticated frameworks are necessary. I will argue that the mental health needs of both sexes are alike, and that attention to sexual difference may distract from important psychological similarities, resulting in discriminatory practice and unjust allocation of resources.

BACKGROUND

It has been argued in recent years that too many women are in prison (Maden et al. 1994, 1996), that many are inappropriately placed in high security (Maden et al. 1995), and that there are insufficient services at lesser degrees of security (Adshead and Morris 1995; Lart et al. 1999).

In 1997, Maden provocatively asked, in relation to forensic services, 'Are women different?' Much new service planning is based on assumptions that women forensic patients are different from their male counterparts. It has been stated that mentally disordered women offenders are characterised by a history of multiple disadvantage, poorly understood mental health problems, inappropriate detention in prison and high levels of distress, masked by antisocial behaviour (Travers 2003). Williams et al. (Chapter 2, this book) note that women offenders commonly have histories of early abandonment and loss, schooling difficulties, and lack of either a stable partnership or a job in their lives. Jeffcote and Travers (Chapter 1, this book) point out that women in secure settings are alienated from their social networks and communities. They also note that the women are both victims and perpetrators of violence, having experienced abuse, usually at the hands of men, during both childhood and adulthood, which has put them at increased risk of mental illness.

Women come to secure services (of whatever level) because professionals perceive them to pose a risk to themselves and/or others. It is well established that women offend much less than men, and proportionately fewer women than men commit violent offences. In high secure settings, women are more likely than men to have been convicted of arson or criminal damage and less likely to have been convicted of interpersonal violence. Among patients admitted to medium security, the number of women who have committed homicide is proportionately greater than the number of men (Coid *et al.* 2000). However, most women who have killed have done so in a domestic context and their placement in a medium rather than high secure setting is likely to reflect the fact that they are perceived to present less of a risk than men to the general public.

In terms of violence to self, repeated and severe deliberate self-harm or self-mutilation is sometimes a reason for women's transfer from prison or general mental health settings to forensic mental health services (Maden *et al.* 1995; Coid *et al.* 2000). However, the study conducted by Coid *et al.* found that referrals to secure services were not triggered by self-harm alone but by self-harm combined with other disturbed behaviour, especially verbal and physical abuse of staff. It is not clear what happens to men who self-mutilate; there are very few of them and, anecdotally, they are equally hard to manage and place.

DIFFERENT FROM WHOM?

It is a central tenet of some accounts of feminist theory that women are defined with reference to men, who constitute a 'norm' because of their assumed social authority. According to this account, women's different experiences, needs and responses are always perceived as 'abnormal' compared with men's. Within forensic mental health services, women do constitute a statistically unusual group, being the numerical minority of patients admitted to secure services. However, they are also unusual when compared with *female* users of general mental health services.

It is very unusual for women to act violently at all; in terms of risk factors for antisocial behaviour, it seems to 'take more' for women to be violent. While it is true that, compared with men, women in secure settings tend to have been convicted of crimes of lesser violence, this should not obscure the fact that a significant group of female patients have acted very violently indeed, in a way that is extremely unusual for women. In addition, arson and criminal damage may represent interpersonal violence even though they do not appear to be interpersonal crimes. Although more women than men enter secure services without a conviction, their admission often follows disturbed behaviour in general mental health settings for which they have not been charged, either because services are reluctant to press charges against patients or because the criminal justice system is reluctant to pursue prosecutions that may fail.

As already noted, intractable self-harming is sometimes seen as needing management in secure settings, but in the minority of women concerned, it is usually accompanied by disturbed behaviour. This combination of self-harm and other disturbance reflects another difference between women admitted to secure settings and other women who use mental health services.

GENDER ROLE STEREOTYPES IN FORENSIC MENTAL HEALTH SERVICES

Feminism argues that sexual differences are often more perceived than real, and arise through the operation of gender role stereotypes, based on prejudice, which in turn can lead to discriminatory practice. Anti-sexist practice, therefore, entails being thoughtful about how, and which, differences are perceived between men and women, and which are given weight in any social system. Sex role stereotypes pervade mental health practice as they do other domains of social life, and forensic mental health services are not exempt. I want to explore some issues of difference between men and women in four areas: work resources, victimisation history, sexual relationships and finally, risk of violence.

Work resources

In the past, women patients were encouraged only to take part in occupations that were identified as 'female' (such as laundry or needlework) while men were offered more 'male' activities (Mezey and Bartlett 1996). However, such overtly discriminating practices are now less common; in general, the more pressing problem about discrimination in terms of access to work experience and rehabilitation is financial. Segregation by sex raises the issue of how to allocate scarce work resources equitably between two services rather than allocating to one. Proper attention to quality and governance issues in mental health care will mean that a service for a small number of patients will either demand a disproportionate share of resources or be vulnerable to closure on the basis that it is not cost-effective. Discrimination may turn out to be financial rather than sexual.

Victimisation history

Nowhere is the question of gender stereotyping more acute than in relation to victim and perpetrator identity. This is a particularly stark issue in both the criminal justice system and forensic mental health services, where victims of crime not only have certain legal rights, but also appear to have additional claims to protection because of their history of injury and hurt. In moral terms of perceived innocence and guilt, perpetrators of harm lose status, and victims gain.

Studies of childhood trauma in patients in secure settings have found high rates of childhood neglect and abuse, both physical and sexual, in both men and women (Heads, Taylor and Leese 1997). Studies in general mental health settings have found high levels of lifetime and childhood victimisation in both sexes (Goodman *et al.* 2001). Longitudinal studies of children who have experienced trauma show that abuse and neglect (especially neglect) are risk factors for personality disorders and substance misuse in adulthood. Childhood traumatic experience is therefore a non-specific risk factor for severe mental illness, substance misuse and personality disorder, all of which are not only common diagnoses in forensic patients but are thought to be functionally linked to the violent behaviour that led to their being admitted to secure settings.

However, the vast majority of childhood victims will not develop severe mental illness or personality disorders and only a minority of those so affected will go on to act violently. The fact of abuse does not itself explain the commission of violence. This is particularly true for women, who in the general population are more likely than men to have suffered some types of abuse or victimisation and yet are clearly not at increased risk of acting violently. Most victims of childhood abuse do not become perpetrators of violence in adulthood; in fact there is some reason to think they avoid such practices (Widom 1994). In women, there is evidence that childhood sexual abuse is a risk factor for only one type of adult criminality: namely, prostitution (Widom and Ames 1994). In contrast, the experience of childhood physical abuse and neglect does seem to be a risk factor for adulthood violence, arrest and psychopathy in men (Luntz and Widom 1994; Weiler and Widom 1996).

Forensic patients are by definition perpetrators of harm and hurt. Some feminist accounts of social violence have also identified violence perpetration as an essentially masculine characteristic; or at least, a characteristic of a particularly toxic kind of masculinity. It may therefore be disconcerting to find this characteristic in women. Given that the majority of victims of violence are female, it is easy to see why femininity is associated with innocent suffering, victimisation, and a type of moral high ground, and why this 'feminine' quality may be hard to detect in male offenders.

The operation of stereotypes can make it hard to acknowledge that male patients have similar histories of childhood abuse to the women, often at the hands of men, and may explain why histories of criminal victimisation are under-reported in men (Newburn and Stanko 1994). If a significant number of women offender patients suffer from undiagnosed and untreated post-traumatic psychological dysfunction as a result of childhood trauma (Zlotkin 1997), then this is also likely to be true of men. Given that some symptoms of post-traumatic stress (especially hyper-arousal and increased sensitivity to threat) increase the risk of violent behaviour, assessing histories of childhood trauma is likely to be important for risk assessment and management with both sexes.

Sexual relationships

Female violence is comparatively so rare that women patients are seen as highly deviant from social norms. Violent and threatening women not only violate ordinary social norms, they also violate sex role and gender role stereotypes of femininity. The fact that they are *statistically* abnormal in terms of behaviour may become confused with their being *sexually* abnormal in terms of behaviour or preferred partners.

Female patients in secure settings may be seen as abnormal if they have relationships with male patients, female patients or nobody at all. In the past, forensic services have been criticised for using crude gender role stereotypes as a measure of mental health. For example, it has been said that female patients were encouraged to have relationships with male patients, as a way of recovering 'normality' (Warner 1996). It is true that it is neither normal nor sensible for a woman to be attracted to a serial rapist; on the other hand, it might be equally true to say that it is not 'normal' for a man to be attracted to an obese arsonist with a long (and evident) history of self-mutilation. What is not explored sufficiently in forensic settings is the meaning of 'normal' sexual relationships for people who have experienced considerable childhood trauma and deprivation, and who are detained in long-term residential settings that are both custodial and therapeutic. Both prison and hospital are social settings in which sexual activity is normally suspended.

Women patients may be at risk from male patients, especially those who have a history of violence towards women. But it cannot be assumed that all male patients are a risk to women, or that they want to have relationships with them. It is possible that male gender role stereotypes about relationships are applied in an unthinking way to male patients; for example, the assumption that all male patients are interested in sexual activity with women and do not discriminate in terms of partner choice. Might this type of gender role stereotyping be a defence against a very painful consideration: that neither the women nor the men in secure settings are attractive to 'normal' people, so they had better get on with each other, because no one else will have them?

The meaning of sexual relationships between patients in secure care is complicated by having to understand these relationships as 'natural' in terms of proximity, as a defence against loneliness, and sometimes as evidence of psychopathology in both parties. These complications are equally true for hetero- and homosexual relationships and for both women and men. We need a much more sophisticated approach to understanding the meaning of sexual relationships between patients, which goes beyond the assumption that men are risky and women are not.

Violence and risk

There have been concerns that because women's violence or cruelty subverts gender role stereotypes, it is easily conceptualised as mental illness (Allen 1987; Mezey and Bartlett 1996). Such a formulation might explain why a greater number of women than men are detained in forensic settings under civil, rather than criminal, sections of current mental health legislation (Maden *et al.* 1995).

Behaviour that violates sex role stereotypes may cause anxiety and aggression from other members of the social group (Cadden 1993). Given that female violence does violate stereotypes, it is sometimes argued that the normal thresholds for assessing risk to self or others (which is the basis for legal detention) are lower for women, and that the behavioural standards for safety, and possible release, are set artificially and unfairly high. Thus risk to self may be used to prevent women's transfer to lower security, and acts of violence or aggression are understood as symptoms of mental illness in women in a way that may not occur in male patients. Presumably, the stereo-type may also work the other way, so that mental disorders are missed in some violent men because their violence is understood as 'normal' mascu-linity.

Violence by women seems to require a special explanation. In contrast, the violence of male patients is often understood as a feature of typical mas-culinity, which does not require further explanation. But any state of mind that can generate violence requires explanation, because it is unusual. Only a minority of men are violent; there is nothing about successful masculinity that predicts violence (Collier 1995). For both men and women, the state of mind that causes violence includes the experience of fear, the wish to be cruel, and the inability to contain anxiety. By assuming that women's violence to others is abnormal, we may be missing out on the common features of violence that a woman offender needs to explore if she is to be safe.

GENDER ROLE IDENTITY IN SECURE SETTINGS

Gender refers to the psychological and social concepts of 'masculine' and 'feminine': how they are constructed, expressed and experienced both by the individual, and their social group. 'Gender role identity' then refers to the process of relating to others as a man or woman; how this is learned and experienced (Notman 1991). An individual of one sex may have much in common with the gender identity of the other, so that a man may feel com-fortable with both a male sex role and some aspects of feminine gender identity. In fact, it is likely that psychological health is associated with a good mix of both masculine and feminine gender identity for both sexes, and a capacity to be flexible about this over time. For example, the concept 'masculine' is commonly associated with independence, dismissal of neediness, assertiveness and strength (see Table 6.1), characteristics that are clearly not confined to men. It would be difficult for *any* adult person to survive a life of work and reproduction without these capacities, and, in reality, both sexes show them in different measure at different times. Hence Freud's famous dictum, that each person brings both masculine and feminine characteristics to his or her relationships with others.

Table 6.1 Psychological characteristics associated with successful masculine and feminine gender identity

Masculinity	Femininity
Assertive/active	Passive/patient
Aggressive	Non-aggressive
Independent	Dependent
Not body conscious	Body defined
Invulnerable	Vulnerable
Reasonable/non-emotional	Emotional/unreasonable
Dismissing of personal neediness	Defined by personal needs
Separate	Connected

It cannot be assumed that male forensic patients are typical of men in general, any more than female patients are typical of women in general. What perhaps is of real concern is that the predominant vision of masculinity on offer to both male and female patients in some high secure settings is a very toxic one, characterised by exploitation of the vulnerable, aggressive denial of dependence and neediness, and physical domination as a determiner of rights. This toxic masculinity stimulates a type of mirroring toxic femininity (see Table 6.2). These are often the only gender roles that are on offer to patients living in secure settings.

There must also be a concern that a dominating, coercive masculinity is the *staff's* principal mode of relating, not only to patients but also to each other in the form of bullying behaviour. Care of patients who have been, and may again be, violent to others involves a degree of imposed control, which may involve shows of strength and the ability to dominate others. Strength and dominance are typically associated with masculine gender identity. It is therefore unsurprising that, for many years, forensic psychiatrists and nurses have usually been male.

Table 6.2 Characteristics of toxic gender identities

Masculine	Feminine
Sadistic: must exert control	Masochistic: permits and provokes control
Attacks and exploits vulnerable	Fails to self-protect
Denies vulnerability in self	Denies destructive cruelty
Idealises strength and conquest	Idealises vulnerability
Denigrates helplessness	Denies agency in self
Defends against grief	Defends against rage
Action not thought	Passive aggressive action
Projects dependence onto others	Provokes rage in others
For both: disparities of power are opportunities for exploitation and cruelty, which is justified by rigid idealisation or denigration.	

It is true, as Travers (2003) says, that women patients are not easily accommodated by current forensic services. But I would suggest that this is to do with the fact that current forensic therapeutic regimes focus extensively on pharmacological interventions. They are massively under-resourced in terms of the psychological interventions that are needed for treatment of complex mental disorders, especially those that are caused by the experience of trauma. Both sexes need safe therapeutic spaces, free from exploitation and harassment, so that they can feel secure enough to do the real work, which is to explore and manage their own capacity for cruelty. If segregation by sex furthers this aim, then it should be pursued. However, if it does not prevent harassment and bullying, and furthermore stretches already thin resources, it may cause more problems than it solves.

CONCLUSION

In the context of developing different services for male and female forensic patients, it is worth considering that one definition of feminism is that no person should be discriminated against on the grounds of either sexual or gender identity. This is not to say that men and women are the same; but rather, that only some differences matter ethically and legally, that differences should not be the basis for abusive or discriminatory practice, and that in terms of human needs and human rights, we are more alike than we are different. Different sub-groups of forensic patients will have different therapeutic needs, but they will be differentiated by a range of psychological, criminological and sociological factors. Physiology and secondary sexual characteristics may be the least, rather than the most, important source of difference.

A colleague of mine (who shall remain genderless) said, somewhat acidly, that the only difference between male and female forensic patients was that women need sanitary towel dispensers in the bathrooms. Perhaps the most problematic gender stereotype at work in forensic mental health services is the belief that men and women's violence is different; so that violence by men is unpleasant, but essentially normal, whereas violence by women requires a special explanation, based on the experience of suffering.

Violence can indeed be a reaction to suffering, but this operates as much for men as it does for women. Violence is what happens when *people* (men and women) are in states of mind characterised by despair and cruelty. In those states of mind, there is rigid polarisation of the good and the bad, denigration of tenderness and vulnerability and an excitement that comes with not caring about anything any more. The aspect of their experience that is most difficult for *all* my patients to talk about in therapy is how much they enjoyed (however briefly) hurting other people.

The crime statistics tell us that for reasons we do not fully understand, more people with Y-chromosomes get into this state of mind than those without. We need, as a matter of social urgency, to find out why more men than women are violent, and to do something about it. Accepting violence as 'boys doing business' is not likely to make things change, and is insulting to those 'boys' who will never be violent. Denying the reality of cruelty in women is not only insulting to women, it is dangerous for all of us.

Acknowledgements

Dr Jackie Short and Dr Gill Mezey provided helpful comments on earlier drafts of this chapter. I am also grateful to Dr Sameer Sarkar for his comments, and for giving me the time to argue with him.

Part II

Practice

Out of this nettle, danger, we pluck this flower, safety.

William Shakespeare
Henry IV, Part I, Act II, Sc. 3, l. II

7

Working Together

Integrated Multi-disciplinary Practice with Women

Tessa Watson, Amanda Bragg and Nikki Jeffcote

INTRODUCTION

This chapter describes a holistic approach to care on a medium secure ward for women. The therapeutic model was developed to provide a way of thinking about and addressing the multiplicity and complexity of the women's needs. It also sought to address the tendency for some women to be offered many interventions while others received almost no therapeutic attention, and to facilitate communication between team members and integration of their work.

ENVIRONMENTAL FACTORS

The restrictive features of a secure ward in a forensic service, and the complex and demanding needs of the women within it, pose constant difficulties in providing the therapeutic opportunities usually taken for granted in less secure and disturbed environments. There may be high numbers of response calls and incidents compared with other wards. Staff turnover is often high, and ward staff can feel under constant pressure in trying to meet the widely varying needs of women with complex presentations, traumatic backgrounds and a diverse mix of symptoms and functional abilities. These difficulties often lead to containment taking priority over therapeutic endeavours, with the result that patients may be unable to realise their potential for progress or recovery.

In an atmosphere of almost continuous crisis management, collaboration and reflection as a team become difficult and often impossible to achieve. Medical and nursing staff tend to feel they carry primary responsibility for containment and physical safety and may see the therapy team's attempts to bring about change as subverting or challenging these priorities. Therapy staff focus on possibilities for new therapeutic sessions, groups and tasks, and may feel these are undermined, blocked or sabotaged by the overriding concern with security. This polarisation results in conflict and a non-therapeutic environment.

In a truly therapeutic environment, the relationship between containment and therapeutic risk is symbiotic. Without safety and containment, therapeutic risk-taking is not possible. Without therapeutic risk-taking, change and progress are limited and women become 'stuck'. As shown in Figure 7.1, this relationship can be portrayed as a continuum, with containment and change at either end of a balance beam, the space between the two points being the zone in which graded assessment, problem-solving and planning can occur.

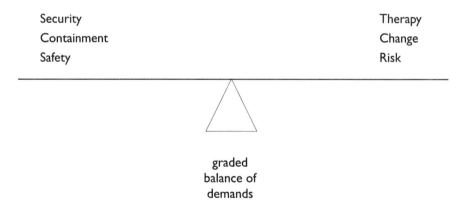

Security   Therapy
Containment   Change
Safety   Risk

graded
balance of
demands

Figure 7.1 Continuum for optimal therapeutic environment

The needs of a particular woman will always be at a point on this continuum. She is more likely to be at the 'containment' end on arrival and will move gradually towards the 'change' end as she progresses towards discharge. However, her position will fluctuate according to her mental state, physical state, life events, losses and goals for treatment. Some women may never move far towards the 'change' end, in which case transfer to a long-term containing environment may become an appropriate goal.

This model of the therapeutic environment mirrors the internal psychological equilibrium of women as conceptualised in attachment theory (see Chapter 1). This highlights the need for a 'secure base', consisting of safe physical boundaries, transparent rules and procedures and good relationships, which a woman can access easily to reduce anxiety at times of stress. When she has regained internal stability and confidence, she can then use the 'secure base' to explore the personal, interpersonal and environmental resources available to her through the facilitating structure of therapeutic relationships and programmes.

The multi-disciplinary team's task is to maximise each woman's therapeutic opportunities and demands whilst also keeping her safe. The balance between security and therapy, containment and change, may vary within an hour, a day, or over longer periods.

IDENTIFYING NEEDS

To identify the needs of the women, a multi-disciplinary needs assessment interview was introduced. This was usually carried out within the first two or three weeks of a woman's admission by the ward psychologist and occupational therapist and the woman's primary or associate nurse. The tone of this meeting was fairly informal, and the focus was on the woman's interests, what she had previously found helpful or unhelpful, and what she wanted in the next few months. Subsequent review interviews, timed to take place shortly before (and to inform) each Care Programme Approach (CPA) meeting, followed a similar format.

Two or three weeks before the CPA meeting, a multi-disciplinary care plan meeting of all professionals involved in the woman's care was held. A schedule of potential areas of need was considered, actual needs were identified and possible ways of addressing them were discussed. The schedule covered the domains identified in standard needs assessment instruments but was expanded and adapted over time to become more gender-specific as the team's experience developed. For example, consideration was given at each meeting to the woman's past experiences of trauma and how these might be re-enacted on the ward; side-effects of medication such as lactation, weight gain and changes in menstrual cycle, and how these might be affecting the woman; body-image and self-esteem; sexual activity and vulnerability; losses and anniversaries; the woman's characteristic ways of dealing with anxiety, distress and anger; and interpersonal issues such as bullying, friendships and attachments to staff. The timing of this meeting allowed for consultation and further information-gathering before the CPA.

CASE EXAMPLES: ANNMARIE, JEMIMA AND JEAN

We now introduce three imagined women in order to illustrate their complex needs, and to suggest the care that they might receive within this therapeutic model. We follow each woman's story from her personal history to her current experience, and discuss treatment aims and care plans that might be agreed upon between her and her care team. For ease of reading we describe the team's input by discipline.

Case example 1: Annmarie

Annmarie's history and current experience

Annmarie is a 25-year-old white Scottish woman who has been on the ward for two years. Detained under Section 3 of the Mental Health Act (1983) (MHA), she has regular unescorted leave. Annmarie has diagnoses of borderline personality disorder, schizo-affective disorder and, occasionally, depression. Previous diagnoses include bipolar affective disorder and schizophrenia. She has a long history of self-harm, including cutting and inserting objects, and has been both anorexic and bulimic in the past.

Annmarie was admitted to secure care after threatening to kill her GP and setting fire to a bin in her hostel. She has a strong attachment to her family (mother, father and four siblings), who have been physically abusive in the past. They visit very infrequently. Annmarie's stepfather may have sexually abused her. Annmarie dropped out of school to care for her siblings in her teens and has since had many inpatient admissions. Her family's Christian religious background has had a strong influence on her. Annmarie experiences confusion around her sexual identity. She lacks close relation-ships, and her friendships are restricted to a few fellow patients. Annmarie has a strong attachment to the ward. She can become close to, and admiring of, particular female members of staff and there have been concerns about possible stalking behaviour. Annmarie sometimes appears to bully more vulnerable women. In all her relationships she swings between appearing childlike or adult-like, making it difficult to judge an appropriate level of leave and responsibility.

Annmarie shows poor impulse control and has difficulty managing her feelings, which can burst out in a chaotic and overwhelming way, or be expressed through self-harm. Annmarie has no conception of her impact on others and says that her outbursts are 'no big deal'.

Annmarie engages sporadically with the therapeutic programme. Her involvement in groups and sessions is either intense or avoidant. She enjoys cooking and crafts, and manages her self-care well. She attends some leisure groups independently.

A lack of single sex hostels, and Annmarie's history of violence and fire-setting, has led to difficulties finding a community placement for her. Episodes of self-harm and violence increase as any discharge plans are developed, leading to a sense of hopelessness in Annmarie and the staff.

Treatment aims

- To reduce episodes of self-harm and work with Annmarie to increase insight into these episodes.

- To develop an understanding of the relationship issues involved in Annmarie's offending behaviour.

- To support Annmarie in developing and maintaining appropriate relationships.

- To consider what service could most usefully meet Annmarie's needs in the long term.

- To support Annmarie in integrating further into her community, with the aim of eventually finding a placement.

Multi-disciplinary care plan

- Medical staff regularly discussed Annmarie's medication and mental state with her. The ward doctor agreed two regular appointment times with Annmarie each week. She encouraged Annmarie to write down her concerns between sessions and to use their appointments to discuss these, rather than repeatedly seeking contact during the week. This helped both Annmarie and the team to understand her thoughts and feelings and the role of medication and relationships in managing them.

- Input from occupational therapists was varied, including planned and unplanned sessions. It included work in the areas of self-care and activities of daily living. The occupational therapist was also able to introduce Annmarie to the physical education instructor and to several gym and aerobics sessions and began to facilitate some community access.

- The ward psychologist provided regular individual sessions to help Annmarie identify realistic and achievable goals in relation to the impulses and experiences that caused her most distress and difficulty. Motivational/commitment work was then carried out for the ward's new dialectical behaviour therapy (DBT) programme, which Annmarie agreed to join. This involved a weekly skills group and twice-weekly individual sessions.

- The arts therapies department offered Annmarie a place in an off-ward mixed sex art therapy group on a regular, weekly basis.

- Annmarie's social worker began to discuss placement possibilities with her. Together, they looked for a supported house, and this also encouraged Annmarie to get to know and use her community. The social worker also made contact with Annmarie's family in order to maintain an open channel of communication.

- Annmarie's primary nurse arranged one-to-one sessions with her regularly and in advance. If the session had to be postponed because of a ward emergency, the primary nurse acknowledged to Annmarie that this was difficult for her and ensured it was immediately rearranged. A DBT skills group was held for a group of ward staff, enabling them to offer Annmarie (and other patients) 'coaching' in DBT skills at times of crisis. The ward psychologist regularly met Annemarie's primary and associate nurses to discuss difficulties encountered by ward staff. Nursing staff monitored Annmarie's weight, her use of as-required medication and her responses to leave, and encouraged a dialogue about these issues.

- When Annmarie self-harmed or behaved aggressively, the team tried to treat this as a temporary setback and focused on helping Annmarie re-orientate to her longer term goals.

- Along with all other women on the ward, Annmarie was invited to attend the weekly women's group.

Outcomes

- There were disagreements among staff about the extent to which Annmarie should take responsibility for dressing her own wounds after self-harm. In addition, the use, at times, of close observations to prevent self-harm was experienced as intrusive by Annmarie and could result in impulsive outbursts. However, over time the overall frequency of her self-harm gradually decreased.

- Annmarie engaged with DBT. She made a commitment to the therapeutic relationship, and became more able to ask for support at times of distress. She was able to 'get back on track' much more quickly after a setback.

- Annmarie was able, with support from nursing and occupational therapy staff, to access services off the ward (including the gym and users' group) and community services (such as swimming and shopping in the community). Annmarie continued occasionally to return from her leave late or to consume alcohol. However, she increasingly came to understand this occurred when she needed more containment, and became more able to seek staff support and to curtail her off-ward activities at these times.

- Annmarie continued to request extra medication, approaching agency staff who were not familiar with her care plan, but this became less frequent.

- Annmarie began to support and help other patients on the ward, although she was still critical and contemptuous of patients and staff at times.

- Four years after her admission, Annmarie and her social worker
  found a small supported women's house, and Annmarie moved
  from the ward. Psychology sessions were increased to help
  Annmarie with the transition and continued on an outpatient basis.

Commentary

The team struggled to keep their focus on treatment rather than management for Annmarie. Her rejection of most therapy groups, and her assertions that 'everything's OK', could lead the team to regard Annmarie's long stay in a secure setting as desirable for her. Her engagement in individual psychology sessions and DBT offered Annmarie and the team an opportunity to consider a future outside secure care.

Annmarie's social worker brought a fresh, 'outside' perspective, reminding Annemarie and the team of the potential for a more normal life in the community.

Annmarie's offending behaviour before her admission was not addressed directly with her. Instead, the threats towards her GP and her fire-setting were formulated as arising from her intense and chaotic emotions, her lack of impulse control and her difficulty in expressing her feelings and needs in words. As she became able to manage her thoughts, feelings and behaviour more effectively, her risk was seen as much reduced.

Staff attitudes towards Annmarie tended to remain polarised. Her progress was sometimes viewed sceptically, and setbacks could be taken as 'proof' nothing had changed. It was hard for the team to remain flexible in the face of Annmarie's fluctuating ability to make choices and decisions. Supervision and support groups for the multi-disciplinary team proved essential in helping staff manage these tensions and differences.

Case example 2: Jemima

Jemima is a 32-year-old mixed-race British woman detained under Section 37/41 of the Mental Health Act. Her diagnosis is schizo-affective disorder with substance abuse, and she suffers with command hallucinations and paranoia. Jemima has burned her arms and chest in the past in response to 'voices', resulting in scarring that has been poorly managed due to inadequate access to primary healthcare. Jemima can be hostile, impulsive and disinhibited, often presents with flat affect and has very low self-esteem.

Jemima had several foster and institutional placements as a child. She will not talk about her childhood, but staff suspect both physical and sexual abuse. She has had numerous psychiatric admissions since the age of 20. Jemima has a history of convictions for acquisitive and minor drug offences. Her index offence involved stabbing a shopkeeper she believed was going to rape her. Jemima has one child, with whom she has no contact. She has had limited contact with her birth parents and values her links with her father's Ghanaian culture.

The secure ward environment enables Jemima to maintain a relatively stable mental state, but as containment and structure are gradually reduced, she decompensates in all areas, often with increased drug abuse. Jemima does not make use of the opportunities available to her on the ward. She isolates herself, often staying in her room, and is reluctant to leave the ward. Jemima finds it hard to make relationships, and is often exploited or exploits others. She is highly ambivalent about engaging in treatment. She experiences mental health services as punitive and controlling and wishes to be free of them. She does not acknowledge any need for support.

Treatment aims

- To enable Jemima to maintain a more stable mental state.
- To help Jemima develop greater awareness of, and responsibility for, her mental state.
- To work with Jemima to understand and address her offending behaviour (including substance misuse).
- To support Jemima in making and maintaining a range of relationships.
- To enable Jemima to access therapeutic and social opportunities, initially on the ward and then outside it.
- To help Jemima develop literacy, numeracy and daily living skills that she had not previously had the opportunity to learn.
- To work with Jemima and her family towards more manageable family relationships.
- To develop a plan for Jemima's future that is acceptable to her.

Multi-disciplinary care plan

- The ward doctor met with Jemima regularly to monitor her medication, mental state and attitudes towards treatment. She gave Jemima information on her illness and began a dialogue with her about how her symptoms contributed to her offence. A referral was made to the general hospital for scar management.

- Jemima was offered individual psychology sessions that built on the ward doctor's work, using a cognitive-behavioural framework for thinking about her psychotic experiences. An assessment of her substance misuse and its function was also carried out, and Jemima was invited to attend a substance misuse group. The opportunity to work with a dialectical behaviour therapy approach was also offered.

- The arts therapies department provided weekly individual music therapy. This aimed to provide Jemima with safe ways of expressing herself, an opportunity to make and maintain a healthy, close relationship, and a containing environment within which to reflect on experiences and feelings.

- The ward occupational therapist offered individual and group sessions. These included work on self-care, self-harm and cultural identity.

- The social worker began a dialogue with Jemima about parenting issues. The legal and practical arrangements involved in renewing contact with her child were explained. Possible future placements were also discussed.

- Jemima was introduced to the education tutor and physical activities co-ordinator by her primary nurse, and was offered the opportunity to take part in education, work rehabilitation and aerobics sessions.

- Jemima's primary nurse offered her frequent sessions without pressuring her to attend. When Jemima was involved in conflict with other patients, whether as perpetrator or victim, this was always discussed with her in a non-judgemental, problem-solving way, either individually or with the other patient. The nursing staff facilitated Jemima's access to the general hospital for scar management.

Outcomes

- Jemima's engagement with staff and with sessions fluctuated considerably. Sometimes she engaged well but would then disengage quickly and unpredictably. She initially seemed curious about a psychological approach to her psychotic symptoms but soon lost interest. The substance misuse assessment suggested she used drugs as a medium for social relationships and to manage her psychotic symptoms, but she would not attend the substance misuse group. She was always ambivalent about DBT and repeatedly stayed in bed at both individual and group session times. She was motivated to cook, and this was facilitated by focusing on dishes that could be prepared without the use of knives.

- Staff noted that changes in environment (including new staff or familiar staff leaving, new patients on the ward or a move of room) frequently triggered a deterioration in Jemima's mental state.

- Jemima began closely supervised and graded contact with her child.

- After a year, the Home Office granted escorted leave for shopping visits in the local town.

- Jemima continued to express dissatisfaction at being on the ward but was also unenthusiastic about high support placements suggested by her social worker.

- Staff explored a referral to the specialist drug and alcohol team but Jemima did not fit their criteria because of her enduring mental illness.

Commentary

The team found Jemima's fluctuating engagement with therapeutic sessions and relationships very difficult to manage. It provoked alternate feelings of hope and hopelessness and staff realised they were blaming themselves, each other and Jemima for her disengagement. The team discussed the importance of Jemima having good role models among the staff. They worked hard to show Jemima healthy, survivable ways of resolving conflict, building respectful relationships and managing emotion. Realising how difficult they themselves found this, particularly at times of high stress on the ward, led to a better understanding of Jemima's difficulties. Staff began to realise how much anxiety and fear of failure or disappointment Jemima experienced. They recognised the need to take advantage of Jemima's times of increased hope, while accepting and supporting her through her hopelessness. However, putting this into practice remained difficult. Some staff carried great anxiety at Jemima's potential for suicide, while others struggled to keep her in mind at all.

Case example 3: Jean

Jean is a 45-year-old white British woman detained under Section 3 of the Mental Health Act, who has recently been admitted following the closure of her long-stay hospital. She has spent over 20 years in inpatient care. Jean's diagnosis is schizophrenia, her first episode of psychosis apparently precipitated by an abusive relationship in which she became pregnant and unwillingly had a termination. Her illness is characterised by thought disorder, persecutory and bizarre ideas and hallucinations. She has a history of chaotic violence and assaultativeness, although she has never been convicted of an offence. She also displays severe behavioural disturbance including stripping, masturbating and faecal smearing in public ward areas. Over the years, Jean has received different treatments including many medications and ECT. Her mood and her hold on reality have, however, continued to fluctuate, with few periods of stability. During Jean's rare episodes of improved mental health, she is calmer, but acutely distressed at her situation.

Jean did well at school and college until her first breakdown. Two of her siblings have very successful careers. Jean has some intermittent contact with her family, but these relationships are not close. Her relatives are often critical of staff when they visit. Staff find Jean likeable but challenging to care for.

Jean can be an intimidating presence on the ward due to her suspicion, bizarre conversation and unpredictable physical presence. She is very isolated and is bullied at times. Jean spends her day restlessly moving around the ward. She has a very disturbed sleep pattern, and is often awake through much of the night. She is not able to engage with any structured activities and rarely feels able to venture away from the ward environment.

Jean's cognitive state is markedly impaired when she is unwell. She finds it hard to manage sustained interactions, and verbal exchanges are often confusing and hard to understand. This makes it difficult to ascertain her intentions and wishes. Jean often neglects her basic physical and environmental care, is often unkempt, smells of urine and has poor skin, with painful sores and rashes.

Jean would like to be on a mixed ward, but in the past she has been highly sexually vulnerable in a mixed environment. The team have been unable to find her the long-term, high support setting she needs.

Treatment aims

- To help Jean settle into the ward environment.

- To work with Jean to improve her quality of life.

- To establish the optimum type and level of medication for Jean.

- To reduce her episodes of distressing behavioural disturbance.

- To explore, with Jean, appropriate placement options.

- To improve Jean's physical health.

- To work with Jean's family in order to build a good relationship between professionals and family members.

Multi-disciplinary care plan

- Nursing and therapy staff planned a careful, staged induction for Jean to the ward environment, key members of staff and treatment opportunities open to her.

- Jean was given a room near an open space where she could move around without disturbing other patients at night.

- Nursing staff provided intensive physical care to improve the condition of Jean's skin and eliminate sores and rashes. They monitored her weight and encouraged her to maintain an adequate diet. Her primary nurse developed a system of unobtrusive but close nursing support when Jean was distressed (particularly at night). Sheets were kept at various places on the ward so that when Jean took her clothes off she could easily be covered without undue fuss. Nursing staff monitored Jean's sleep pattern and encouraged her to stay up for longer in the day and retire at night. She was encouraged to drink herbal teas and to reduce her fluid intake in the evening to prevent night-time incontinence. Staff facilitated access to the garden and grounds, with unobtrusive escorts. Jean was also helped to access dental and chiropody services, on the ward where possible.

- Medical staff undertook detailed research into Jean's medication history and carefully considered the options. Changes were explained to Jean simply, at times when she was more settled. 'Well woman' issues were also addressed with her.

- The psychology department allocated one member of staff to work with Jean. The psychologist first initiated ad hoc contact with Jean. Over a period of months this developed into a regular appointment, which Jean could use as she wished.

- Jean was offered a slow and gradual introduction to a member of staff from the arts therapies department. Jean expressed an interest in working with drama, and began to develop a therapeutic relationship with the dramatherapist attached to the ward. Two 20 minute sessions were offered to Jean each week. Initially these took place on the ward, but as a therapeutic alliance was developed, the dramatherapist offered Jean the opportunity to use the off-ward dramatherapy room. After a gradual four-month introduction to the space, the sessions were transferred to this room. She was also invited to join the music therapy group which ran each week on the ward.

- The occupational therapist offered Jean varied opportunities for individual work including work on self-care, self-image, and education around healthy eating and weight. The therapist worked with Jean to help her use a journal or diary, which enabled her to maintain a greater sense of continuity and to remember happenings on the ward. Jean was introduced to the sensory room and began to use this extensively as a way of calming and soothing herself. When Jean's mental state allowed, the therapist took brief opportunities to support Jean in community access to the local park.

- The social work department made contact with Jean's family and developed an ongoing, supportive relationship. This enabled Jean's family to maintain contact with her even when it was too distressing for them to visit. The social worker also discussed possibilities for a future placement with Jean and her family.

Outcomes

- Jean built relationships with staff extremely slowly, but these were maintained. She communicated the importance of her relationships with her primary nurse, occupational therapist, psychologist and dramatherapist. Jean became very distressed when the occupational therapist said she would be leaving, and careful planning was undertaken to say goodbye and remember the important work that had been done.

- Jean's family were able to maintain regular contact and their anger towards the service lessened.

- Staff found caring for Jean traumatic at times, especially when they had to restrain her and witnessed her profound fear and distress. Attempts to obtain agreement for an all-female response team for patients like Jean were not successful.

- Jean made increasing use of the sensory room, gradually asking to go there on her own or with a member of staff. She was in this way able to take some control over her distress.

- Jean's mental state continued to fluctuate. Funding could not be agreed for the one high-support home found by the social worker.

Commentary

Providing and maintaining a therapeutic environment for Jean was a constant challenge for staff. During her most distressed phases Jean would damage and destroy property and become incontinent. Constant repair and replenishment of Jean's basic environment was an exhausting task. However, staff persisted in maintaining a nurturing environment for Jean and avoiding a punitive approach. The ward manager resisted pressure arising from the expense of cleaning Jean's carpet to replace it with linoleum. Staff shared the task of supporting Jean, to avoid the emotional and physical demands involved falling only on her primary nurse.

Therapists discovered that initially their input needed to be highly flexible for Jean to be able to take opportunities for contact. The environment for such meetings was also important and it was essential to have quiet spaces, both on and off the ward, that could be used without pre-booking.

The team found it hard to see that Jean was making any progress and this was experienced as demoralising. Gathering detailed information that would be of help to a new placement helped staff to feel they were planning for Jean's future.

Jean had suffered many losses and staff often felt that she was expressing her grief in her behaviour. Supervision and support for staff with these intense emotional experiences was essential.

CONCLUSION

A number of common themes run through each of these women's stories and we finish by summarising them.

Time

Women need time to build relationships with staff and to be able to engage with treatment and activities. A slow, graded introduction to new staff and environments is useful. A trusted member of staff can introduce the woman to a new therapist or take her to a new session, and withdraw support gradually. Without this, women may feel that new relationships and opportunities are not manageable.

Relationships

Women are highly sensitive to their social environment and need the consistency and predictability that has often been lacking in their lives. Staff departures need to be acknowledged to give a chance for feelings to be addressed, and the increased stress for women at times of change or uncertainty should be taken into account in teams' expectations and planning.

Specialist needs

There is often a need to seek specialist input, for example, by involving drug and alcohol or learning disability teams. The boundaries between different agencies can be hard to negotiate and women with complex needs often fall between services. In some settings, the development of specialist worker posts might enable a greater ease of access to expertise and to the services of outside agencies.

Flexibility

Each woman moves within a continuum of mental health. The fluctuations and changes in her mental state may follow a pattern or be unpredictable. This is distressing for the woman, and presents challenges to the multi-disciplinary team, who need to be able to moderate support, treatment and security to offer useful care in a consistent way. An appointment-based, structured programme, or therapist-led agenda, will not be accessible to all women. Staff need to be flexible and responsive, offering a range of approaches, to help women engage as well as they can at any given time.

Ward spaces and environments are often not conducive to therapeutic endeavours. A flexible, safe environment is needed with a range of spaces for both regular and unplanned, formal and informal contact.

Staff support

Effective work with women requires close communication and support between team members. Staff may experience feelings of hope, despair, hostility, affection, pity, anxiety, anger and fear, and will at times come under pressure to respond unthinkingly, punitively and dismissively. Formal and informal support and supervision are needed to help both individuals and teams deal with these experiences and avoid unresolved conflicts, splitting and burnout.

8

Thinking under Fire

The Challenge for Forensic Mental Health Nurses Working with Women in Secure Care

Anne Aiyegbusi

INTRODUCTION

Providing effective nursing care for women detained in secure mental health services is a challenging and complex task. The needs of women patients are frequently extensive and it may be tempting to overlook the difficulties encountered by nurses who attempt to work with this patient group. Traditional nursing models are likely to be only partially effective. It is safe to say that interventions shown to be effective with less interpersonally disturbed populations may be experienced as persecutory or provocative by many women who find themselves detained in secure mental health services. Care is frequently difficult to provide because of this. For nurses, working in these environments is often highly stressful. In particular, the emotional impact on nurses can be severe. In the absence of sufficiently robust frameworks with which to make sense of the intense emotional content of interpersonal contact, there is a high risk of nurses becoming drawn into toxic relationships with the women patients, other professional groups and each other.

I will suggest in this chapter that unless the emotional impact of working in secure services for women is addressed in an effective way, nursing interventions to address clinical needs are difficult to implement. The danger is that, rather than an effective treatment service, a toxic environment develops where care and treatment play second fiddle to painful conflict and acrimony. I will discuss the value of a psychodynamic perspective for making sense of the intense emotional communications that underpin much of the emotional hard labour involved in working as a nurse in women's secure services. Because there is a dearth of research into the nursing care of women in secure services, much of the material I will present in this chapter has been derived from ten years of clinical nursing experience in this area.

CASE EXAMPLE 1

Repeated problems have been experienced in a secure mental health unit for 18 women patients. These problems include a high level of incidents including self-injury, breaches of security on the part of patients and staff, verbal abuse, and physical assault by patients on each other and on nursing staff. Staff sickness and turnover is very high, meaning that it is commonplace to have temporary staff working on the unit. Morale is very low and the unit has a bad reputation within the wider service for being an unpleasant place to work. The fact that six of the patients have been nursed under continuous observations for a protracted period of time without any signs of improvement adds to nurses' low morale. Some nurses feel the patients get too much of their own way while others feel the patients are suffering because they are disempowered and treated too harshly. Managers' impressions are of a unit in chaos but various attempts to address the difficulties have been unsuccessful. That the unit has had five different managers in the past two years is seen as a major contributory factor.

Relationships between multi-disciplinary team members are problematic with many nurses seen as unprofessional and unable to meet the needs of the patients due to poor training and little understanding of the patients' complex needs. The nurses feel the wider multi-disciplinary team fail to appreciate how difficult the patients are, and that they regularly side with patients against nurses. The nurses are particularly aggrieved because they feel their multi-disciplinary colleagues believe everything the patients say without reference to the nursing view of events. However, the nurses are struggling within their group because of bullying and the formation of different 'cliques' who cannot work together, each group feeling that their approach to patient care and management is the right one. Gossip, aggressive practical jokes and general undermining of each other is commonplace.

Discussion

The above case example is typical of many secure services for women at one time or another. A psychodynamic framework offers one way of making sense of the chaos and disturbance that blights women's secure mental health services. Davies (1996) has explained how professionals working in forensic services may be drawn into the internal world of the offender. He makes the following observation:

> The view is taken that professionals who deal with offenders are not free agents but potential actors who have been assigned roles in the individual offender's own re-enactment of their internal world drama. The professionals have the choice not to perform but they can only make this choice when they have a good idea what the role is they are trying to avoid. Until they can work this out, they are likely to be drawn into the play, unwittingly and therefore not unwillingly. Because of the latter, if the pressure to play is not anticipated, then the professional will believe he is in the role of his choosing. (Davies 1996, II p.133)

Following Davies' formulation, the disturbance characterising secure services for women may be understandable when the patients' internal worlds are taken into consideration.

TRAUMATIC INTERNAL WORLDS

It is well documented that women mentally disordered offenders as a group have experienced high levels of early abandonment, rejection, loss and abuse (Department of Health 2002a). Women in secure mental health services will therefore have experienced high levels of trauma in their early caregiving relationships. Adshead (1998) explains how 'maladaptive' behaviours engaged in by some disturbed psychiatric patients can be understood as traumatic re-enactments of early rejection and abuse by primary caregivers. Because of their developmental antecedents, women in secure care are likely to present a number of challenges to nursing staff, whose role it is to provide care in the context of the nurse-patient relationship. The maladaptive behaviour of women patients may be related to nurses' attempts to provide care. Intolerable fear and anxiety is provoked in the patients, who anticipate the pain of rejection or perverse behaviour on the part of caregivers, based on their prior experience. One strategy to manage anxiety is to corrupt or destroy the relationship in a kind of pre-emptive strike before the nurse has a chance to reject, abandon or abuse. Another strategy involves applying interpersonal pressure to the nurse until she or he acts in a way similar to the way previous caregivers have behaved. This also functions to reduce anxiety because the patient will be familiar with the type of relationship she has now created with the nurse, no matter how unsatisfactory.

The extreme behavioural disturbances of many women in secure care include those that are self-directed, involving acts of self-injurious behaviour, and those that are directed outwards in the form of violence or verbal abuse. These behaviours are difficult to manage in an inpatient setting. The difficulties involved in managing behavioural disturbance are compounded when groups of these women reside together, due to the emotional environment created. Primitive defence mechanisms, such as splitting, projection and projective identification are unconsciously employed to manage the anxiety aroused by being placed on the receiving end of care. The emotional impact associated with working with the patients may be explained by these dynamics. When professionals are unable to contain these powerful processes, acting out on their part is pre-dictable. As Davies puts it, professionals will be compelled to act out roles unconsciously ascribed to them by the patients unless they know what those roles are. It is therefore important to understand the patients' internal world dramas. In this respect, the psychological effects of early trauma and failed care provide a template against which we may make sense of patients' current presentations.

MAKING OTHERS SUFFER

Women patients in secure care are not only victims but make others suffer too. Whether charged with or convicted of a criminal offence, detention in a secure unit is mostly determined by interpersonal violence, fire-setting or repeatedly breaking rules in less secure services to the extent that risk to others is increased. The need to make others suffer may be a strategy for managing unprocessed pain, or in other words, pain that cannot be thought about. This may involve feelings associated with past victimisation, including anger, exposure, humiliation, rejection, shame, intrusion, being dehumanised and being powerless to the will of a perpetrator. These feelings are unbearable and yet they are part of the patient's life experience and central to understanding her current predicament. While some women may keep repeating the experience of being victimised in relationships, others need to make somebody else feel their pain. Most women detained in secure mental health services are likely to flip between these two states of mind. This 'flipping' underpins the propensity to be both victim and perpetrator of interpersonal distress. A clinical example would be a woman patient who repeatedly injures herself, while emotionally abusing the nurses who are tasked with providing care for her. The relationships many of the women form include a victim and a perpetrator and so the patients bully and victimise each other. In many units there will be a pecking order where those at the bottom are exploited materially and emotionally by the 'top dogs'. Property, food, prescribed medication, shopping or any other asset is seemingly fair game. Here, the sense of being repeatedly robbed is likely to be among the distressing states of mind that are being projected from one person and forced into another. Patients who are being bullied often remain in a deteriorated state, forcing staff input for protection from other patients as much as for clinical reasons.

Unbearable feelings that cannot be processed mentally are projected onto others. For example, when a patient engages in self-injurious behaviour, nurses who discover her actions may feel intensely angry, frightened, powerless and exposed. Thus, the self-injuring patient who is unable to think about or communicate verbally the overwhelming feelings that led to her behaviour, has in fact communicated by impact (Casement 1985). She has communicated by making somebody else feel what she is feeling but cannot process mentally. Many women detained in secure mental health services communicate their intolerable affects through the counter-transference. This may explain the intense and negative emotional atmosphere that can prevail in secure services for women where groups of individuals with similar psychopathologies reside together.

CONTAINMENT

In psychoanalytic psychotherapy, the process whereby a patient projects intolerable parts of the self into the therapist is a well-understood mechanism and is of value therapeutically. For nurses who are also used by patients as receptacles for intolerable parts of the self, there may not be a framework for making sense of the experience. Likewise, there may be no established model for turning the experience into something positively therapeutic for the patient. As Hinshelwood (1994) points out, the psycho-analyst contains the patient's projections as a way of helping the patient to begin to understand this part of the self. By holding on to the projection, the psychoanalyst demonstrates that the intolerable affect can in fact be thought about. When the patient is better able to think about the projection, the psychoanalyst begins to feed it back in a way the patient can manage. Bion (1959) warns that if the analyst fails to contain the patient's projection and forces it back into the patient, it is experienced as even more painful than before.

Although containment is in many ways a psychoanalytic or psychodynamic concept, it is a critical component of the task forensic mental health nurses are required to undertake in their work with very disturbed women patients. Failure to contain the patients' projections is likely to lead to even more distress on the part of patients while causing dis-turbance in the staff group. For example, a woman patient who, because of her past experiences of rejection and abandonment, is overwhelmed with anxiety about engaging in yet another relationship with a professional carer, may verbally abuse her new primary nurse. The initial task of the new primary nurse is then to contain the patient's fear and anger. The danger is that the new primary nurse acts out on the feelings the patient has projected and, as a result, rejects her. This would be a re-enactment of the patient's past trauma, with the new primary nurse having been drawn into acting out a script from the patient's internal world drama.

Projective identification is a term that describes the process of acting out a patient's projections. This powerful and primitive defence mechanism is particularly difficult to manage for nurses working with groups of patients who employ it in an intense way. There is constant pressure to act out and when containment is not understood, and skills to think under fire have not been developed, then acting out by professionals is exactly what will happen. Nurses are based primarily in the patients' social environment, they work in close proximity to the patients for protracted periods of time and their main therapeutic tool is the nurse-patient relationship. As I have mentioned before, the risk is that nurses are drawn into re-enactments of the patients' early traumatic experience with primary caregivers.

TOXIC ENVIRONMENTS

Patients are trying to live with overwhelming emotional pain and project this into staff through various communications such as self-injury, very direct sexualised communications, physical assaults and vicious personalised verbal attacks. The unconscious hope is that the nursing staff can do something positive with the communication, in particular that they can at least use it to understand what the patient is feeling. However, containment such as this requires nurses to be able to think while under extreme pressure to act in response to the distress that has been forced into them. The risk is that, in shock, nurses lash back at the patients and therefore re-enact rejection and abusive interactions. A further risk is that instead of processing, nurses act out within the staff group so that communication between colleagues is hurtful. This includes bullying, aggressive practical jokes, gallows humour, gossiping and backbiting. Gender differences provide a natural split and an opportunity for toxic interactions. Unprocessed material emanating from the patients' histories can become part of the unwritten agenda from which professional men and women relate with each other. Emotionally hurtful sexual liaisons and rage at male perpetration of abuse can be seen as flip sides of the same coin in terms of serving as defences against the painful histories of abuse the women patients present with.

Staff may launch envious attacks on colleagues who are receiving support or training. This is likely to reflect emotional deprivation in the staff group. Cox (1996) refers to the way staff in a special hospital can be '…hungry – but not for food. They can be hungry for confidential supervision at an appropriate depth' (II p.447). It is through regular supervision and other opportunities to reflect on clinical work that nurses learn to contain patients' projections. Importantly, the sense of receiving sensitive, supportive input, whether through supervision, teaching or staff support, may reduce nurses' anxieties about being left in an intolerable situation by management, who may be experienced as uncaring parents.

Of course, not all the disturbance in a women's secure service can be a result of the patients' psychopathologies. Hinshelwood and Skogstad (2000) explain how the unconscious material nurses bring to their work can have the effect of undermining containment. It is for this reason that self-awareness is of critical importance for nurses who work with women in secure mental health services.

AN ATTACHMENT THEORY APPROACH

Attachment theory is based on the seminal work of Bowlby (1951) who studied the emotional impact on children of being separated from their primary caregivers and found that lack of maternal love laid the foundations for disturbance in mental health and personality. Bowlby's work unfolded into a theoretical framework called attachment theory. Because attachment theory regards relationally disturbed behaviours as a function of emotional insecurity within a caregiving/care-receiving relationship, it may be an effective framework for forensic mental health nurses to apply in their clinical work with women patients who have experienced failed early care.

CASE EXAMPLE 2

Jasmine is the fifth child of a woman who was consistently described as having chronic and severe problems with alcohol abuse. All of Jasmine's elder siblings had, at some stage in their childhood, been taken into the care of the local authority due to neglect and cruelty by both of their parents. Jasmine was removed from her parents into local authority care at the age of three months due to neglect. She was observed at the time to be floppy and malnourished. After spending time in a paediatric unit, she was placed with foster parents.

At six months of age, Jasmine was adopted. At 18 months of age she was again admitted to a general hospital where she was found to be suffering from malnutrition. In addition she was noted to be infested with head and body lice, and had several old bruises about her body suggestive of physical assault. She was returned to local authority care. At six years of age, Jasmine was again fostered but was soon returned to institutional care because her foster parents found her to be unmanageable. She remained in institutional care for the remainder of her childhood.

By the time Jasmine was 14 she was repeatedly violent, self-injurious and socially alienated. She was engaging in petty criminality and was also lighting fires and so was admitted to secure accommodation. Just before Jasmine's seventeenth birthday, she set fire to the dormitory of the secure unit, claiming that it was her intention to escape while the building was being evacuated. After spending a short period of time on remand, Jasmine was transferred to a secure psychiatric service with a diagnosis of borderline personality disorder. Her behavioural disturbance increased. She repeatedly harmed herself and, during the subsequent interventions by nursing staff, frequently lashed out, stating that she did not want her wounds dressed. Jasmine spent a great deal of time in seclusion during the early part of her admission and the care team felt at a loss as to how to provide care and treatment. Additionally, it was soon identified that Jasmine had a profound eating disorder. She claimed not to want food and rarely ate.

Discussion

Jasmine's earliest attachment was characterised by abuse perpetrated by her primary caregiver. By the age of three months, it could be inferred from the available case information that she had failed to internalise a basic sense of security and of her own worth in terms of expecting her needs for care and protection to be met. By experiencing a continual change of caregivers Jasmine had failed to expect continuity of care, another basic ingredient of psychological security. She experienced loss which, at such an early age, would have been processed as a form of psychological trauma (de Zulueta 1993). By 18 months of age, Jasmine had learned that the vulnerability associated with dependency is met with pain, humiliation and rejection. This will have prohibited her from bonding with anyone, especially those tasked with her care. The experience of long-term institutionalisation during childhood and adolescence compounded her predicament due to lack of opportunity to have her expectations disconfirmed by a positive, secure, caregiving attachment figure. Jasmine's disturbed behaviour and criminality during adolescence could be understood as a function of the psychological, biological and social consequences of repeated trauma and failed attachment. Fonagy et al. (1997) observe that during adolescence, attachment to parents or primary caregivers is temporarily transferred to groups and institutions during the ordinary developmental challenge posed by adult individuation. Accordingly, when attachment has been compromised by early experience with caregivers, its abnormalities become increasingly conspicuous during teenage years in the form of a developmental surge in criminality.

Attachment-oriented care

An attachment-oriented approach was taken to Jasmine's care and treatment. This involved focusing on her relational behaviour and understanding it as stemming from her prior experience of being vulnerable and in need of care. As a fundamental principle, it was understood that staff would aim to disconfirm Jasmine's maladaptive expectations of relationships with carers, while recognising that Jasmine's behaviour could be perpetuated if current caregivers responded in a reciprocal manner. Jasmine's attacks on offered care were understood as a consequence of her unconscious expectation that the offer of care would be followed by abuse, humiliation and the pain of rejection and loss. It was also understood that Jasmine had no coherent internal model of how her needs for care could be met and so could not imagine what this would be like.

The initial aim was to achieve a therapeutic alliance with Jasmine. This involved, in the first instance, establishing a positive rapport between Jasmine and her carers. A small team of professionals was allocated to meet Jasmine's needs for care and treatment. It was understood that, given Jasmine's attachment history, it was unlikely that she would establish a secure relationship with an individual caregiver. Through previous experience it had been found counter-productive to expect any individual to manage the degree of relational disturbance present in a person with Jasmine's attachment history and current presentation. The intensity of the 'special' relationship that inevitably unfolded in such cases would hold a high risk of burnout for the individual caregiver and a repeat of prior abandonment for Jasmine. Both parties, it was predicted, would be likely to end up alienated by such a strategy. Therefore, a small team consisting of ward-based nurses, a therapist and psychiatrist worked together in implementing a collaborative care plan. This approach had been explained to and agreed by Jasmine, who recognised that she was not ready to rely on any individual person.

Central to the care plan was a consistent approach. Jasmine had been asked how she felt about contact with professionals. She initially denied that she had any need for clinical input, stating that she just wanted to be left alone. However, it was noted that Jasmine's periods of self-injury tended to occur when members of nursing staff were occupied with other patients' needs. This suggested that Jasmine did desire contact with carers and became unsettled when she saw available care directed at other patients. This hypothesis was discussed with Jasmine who eventually agreed that she did not feel safe when there were no nurses around. However, she said that she felt overwhelmed with panic and anger when she felt nurses were crowding in on her. As a way forward, it was agreed that nurses would communicate their availability and willingness to support Jasmine by frequent, short contacts asking how she felt and stating that they were there should she need anything. Jasmine said she found this helpful. Jasmine's therapist met with her regularly and focused on developing a sense of attunement, learning to understand how Jasmine felt and feeding this back to her. For example, if Jasmine complained of experiencing many urges to self-injure during the previous week, her therapist would suggest that this might be a way that Jasmine had learned to deal with her internal pain. Jasmine came to understand the extent of her internal pain and that for many years she had tried to block this out with self-injury.

Jasmine's small team worked together, sharing new information about Jasmine so that they could ensure consistency and a common language with which to approach and address Jasmine's day-to-day needs. Over a period of months, they did establish a positive, therapeutic rapport with Jasmine who was less distressed by the thought of relationships with carers. This was evident in a reduction in her self-harm and in the length of time she spent isolated in seclusion. Jasmine commented on the fact she is beginning to trust her care team and understands that they are trying to help her. Rather than behaving in a way that automatically pushes carers away, Jasmine is beginning to approach her team of carers when she feels they could help her.

CONCLUSION

Women receiving care and treatment in secure environments present with a complex range of needs that are hard to meet. For nurses, this complexity is made especially challenging both by the nature of the nursing role and by the fact that their main therapeutic tool is the nurse-patient relationship. Anxiety based on early trauma with caregivers is stirred up in the patients.

The only means patients have of communicating their distress may be to make nurses who care for them suffer emotionally. However, if nurses can learn to contain the patients' projections, therapeutically meaningful work can take place. This can be achieved only when nurses are afforded effective supervision and therefore opportunities to think about their interactions with patients within a supportive and containing structure.

Attachment theory offers a framework for understanding emotional and behavioural disturbance within caregiving/care-receiving relationships and for helping nurses increase patients' internal sense of security within the nurse-patient relationship. Once a patient's emotional security has been increased through containment, other interventions to address her clinical needs are more likely to be sustained.

9

Hiding and Being Lost

The Experience of Female Patients and Staff on a Mixed Sex Ward

Anna Motz

Looking around the daily community meeting one morning I was struck by the fact that of the seven women on this mixed, long-term low secure ward, six of them were, or seemed to be, hiding. One remained in her room, escaping the tension, drama and conflict offered by this meeting. Three others had placed themselves in corners of the room. One crouched down, close to the ground. Another stood, arms folded, against the door and the last sat behind the circle of chairs, making herself virtually invisible, although she was still nominally present in the room. Only one sat in the circle, but she avoided eye contact altogether, and spoke only when addressed directly.

I was put in mind of the children's game of peek-a-boo, where the child delights in losing and finding the mother's face, and of hide-and-seek. Hide-and-seek allows the hiders the experience of fleeing, exciting and fearful, and hiding, safe in the expectation of being found. The seekers have the lonelier and more persecutory task of hunting down the hiders. I resisted my strong urge, both maternal and predatory, to draw those hiding female patients from their secret places, to collect them up and place them in the circle, to be seen.

In this chapter I will look at the experience of female patients on a mixed ward, as mirrored in the feelings of the professionals who work with them. I will point out the sense in which the hide-and-seek motif characterises the interactions between the women and the workers and illustrates the central conflict for women with a severe personality disorder: the desire for intimacy, and to be known, understood and helped, in constant battle with the wish to defend themselves against this contact and remain isolated and at war. How are staff members to work with this paradox? And how to begin to address the reflected split in this staff group as they struggle with the desires to help, contain and comfort, conflicting with the equally strong urges, at times, to abandon, disappoint and retaliate against these women?

One of the central features of women with severe personality disorders is their conflicted, ambivalent and frightened relationship with others and with themselves. The fear of being seen, literally because of shame and fear of sexual assault, and figuratively as a metaphor for being known, is reflected in their hiding, curling up and making themselves invisible. I think this relates to a central conflict between the wish for privacy, to be left alone, and the fear of total isolation and abandonment. The desire for closeness is in powerful conflict with the fear of intimacy.

HIDING AND SHAME

For many women with severe personality disorders their feminine body is lost, covered, hidden under baggy clothing, layers of flesh, scars, hair falling in the face, piercings, tattoos. The sexual body has often been the site of abuse and violation, and so an attempt is made to cover it up, disguise and transform it. It may also become the site of embodied trauma and protest, as I will discuss when I look more closely at the phenomenon of self-harm.

The naked body is often covered up completely, and the most obviously recognisable feminine aspect is often that of the girl, in childish jewellery, kittens on tee shirts, socks, and slippers. This can be encouraged by staff, whose maternal feelings become activated by their awareness of deprivation in these patients' early lives. There may also be a paternalistic and infantilising culture of care for women with severe personality disorders. I have often been struck by the sense in which the barren and severe aspect of special hospitals, with their high walls and secure fences, are softened internally by the abundance of stuffed animals, which are scattered throughout the rooms of female patients. It could be suggested that this type of infantilising is a defence by the staff against recognition of the violence and adult sexuality of such patients. Instead of attributing adult functioning to these women, they are stripped of their competence and the staff's own vulnerable, childlike and needy feelings are projected into them. This type of splitting and projection is an example of a defence against the overwhelming anxiety of working closely with women in so much pain, with such profound levels of disturbance.

The pain of their adult lives is often lost in an environment that disguises it by failing to remember their histories, particularly the most traumatic aspects. 'Losing' the memories of abuse and trauma that the women have experienced also seems to reflect an unconscious defence against overwhelming anxiety. This process again leaves the patients hidden. The environment seems to be designed to block out and cover up the psychic reality these women face now and have borne in their past. These defences, engaged in by staff of all disciplines, but particularly those who are in closest contact with the patients, the nurses, are codified in the culture of these institutions, which often provide no thinking spaces where practice can be analysed and understood.

At times the women can be seen but not heard. They are not only hidden but also silenced. In the mixed ward, the male patients choose to play loud music much of the time, drowning out conversation in the communal areas. I am struck by the loud, often romantic and sentimental music that plays in the unit, its lyrics jarringly at odds with the scene in which they are played. For example, to a group of isolated, dishevelled women with no sense of being attractive or loveable: 'You're gorgeous, I would do anything for you.'

As the title of this paper suggests, the situation of the women on this mixed ward is not only that they are lost within the system, sometimes out of a kind of wilful forgetting, but also that they hide themselves away. There is an important sense in which these women have chosen to hide, perhaps out of a desire for privacy, safety and some kind of dignity. I want to suggest that another powerful motivation is their profound sense of shame about the events that have shaped their lives, about their current situations, about their involvement in shameful activities; and about their rage, which they would love to discharge. This shame results in the need to avoid being seen. As Gilligan (1999) suggests in his study of violence, the look of the 'other' is crucial to the concept of shame. It is as if by hiding they cannot be seen; a type of magical thinking. Another form of magical thinking may also be at work as the women avoid our gaze, like infants who think that if they close their eyes they are invisible to us. They may hold the unconscious belief that if they look away or hide their eyes, they cannot be seen. They can be invisible, unchallenged, and left alone, their shame not exposed.

WHAT HAS BEEN LOST? WHAT IS HIDDEN?

If shame is the motivation for hiding, it becomes essential for us, staff working with these women, to gain some understanding of what it is that creates this sense of shame and loss. These women have lost their sense of identity within their families, peer groups, and wider society. Crucially, they may feel bereft of their cultural identity, which seems particularly difficult to preserve in the ward environment. There is often a loss of racial identity and a sense of blending into a homogenous group of 'patients' who are without individual features. For many black women this type of merging into white culture may feel profoundly uncomfortable and evoke a deep sense of betrayal and loss.

For many of these women the ordinary experiences of womanhood have been destroyed or perverted. Their hidden losses may include miscarriages, stillborn children, adopted children or even murdered children. Their sense of themselves as part of the community of women, as mothers, has been destroyed, as has their sense of reproductive capacity and mothering possibilities. In the unit where I work, with only one exception, the losses and burdensome secrets include the early, traumatic loss of sexual innocence, through incest or extra-familial abuse.

ENVY AND CURIOSITY: THE IMPACT ON STAFF

The women often comment on us, female staff – what we look like, whether we have children – with a kind of resigned admiration that may well disguise envy, but which in any case highlights the sense of shared gender but totally different experience of femininity. This can create strong feelings in all staff, particularly feeding into narcissistic needs for gratification or, alternatively, into our fears about being found, or even found out. The idealisations and desire to know about us may be both flattering and frightening, making *us* want to hide away.

The potential for identification with these women may itself be a threatening prospect, inviting us to imagine what it might be like to be in their situation. I believe that this dynamic is particularly powerful for women working as therapists and nurses with women with severe personality disorders. Confronting our own fears of going mad, of losing children and our sense of self-worth, as well as having major restrictions placed on our sexual, physical and psychic freedom, is a truly frightening prospect. Defending against such an identification requires strategies for distancing oneself, which may include an angry withdrawal or a disavowal of affinity that is an attempt to split off unacceptable fears or impulses and locate them in the women patients, perceived largely as 'other'.

CASE EXAMPLE 1: LOSS, MOURNING AND 'CONFUSEMENT'

The events I am about to describe took place in the weekly women's group on the ward, itself an attempt to create a safe and enclosed setting for the women on the unit. In one group there was an intimate discussion of the losses of children, and how devastating it would be for anyone outside the hospital to hear about these experiences, how impossible to accept and understand. The women in the group were very split in their relation to their losses. One had become mute with grief, and related like a child herself, rocking and smiling, offering us sweets. Several patients gave the impression of being children in foster care, being offered apparent kindness but feeling they had to pay their way, making sure we, the staff, were placated and 'bought' with sweets and expressions of gratitude.

Another woman, a fire-setter of long standing, found the experience of being in a more intimate setting than the ward both distressing and welcome at the same time. She became so confused and angry that she mixed up her words as she attempted to describe her experience, remembering how she had been talked into the decision to let her son be adopted, saying how the nurses had 'defused' her. She went on to describe her overwhelming sense of 'confusement', which seemed a composite concept of confusion, debasement and de-fusion, that is, being left with no potency or hope.

This arsonist spoke of being 'defused' by staff, evoking an image of a bomb having its force, its dangerousness, removed. She viewed this as a kind of stripping of her power, a humiliating and painful process. Staff in turn described her as having 'burned out the nurses'. This, to me, as in so many parallel cases, expressed clearly the dynamics of projective identification in which she had split off and projected her anger and despair so powerfully that it had been located in the nursing staff, who, in turn, had been 'burned out', destroyed by the experience of intense rage. She was no longer left with the anger, but had evacuated it into those around her, and was left, if anything, empty. Her experience of being 'defused' may have reflected this process, which I would argue had taken place at an unconscious level. A nurse's understanding of how this rage had been projected into her, enacted in her angry attempts to control this patient, and then burned through her, was conveyed when she said 'She burns us out.' Something of the relentlessness and force of the patient's experience and psychopathology is conveyed through this description.

A third woman, who had taken a baby some 15 years ago, for which she had spent 11 years in a special hospital, seemed to have taken on the role of articulating the pain of mourning, and she spoke about losses with candour and sadness. Losses of children, privacy, identity, hope and sexual dignity were common experiences. This discussion led to a sharing of feelings of vulnerability and violation, particularly in relation to the men on the unit, with their sexually predatory and disinhibited behaviour.

Within the group setting the staff seemed able to relate to and contain these feelings, but on the ward there was little sense of understanding. The traumatic experiences were kept at a distance, and the emotional impact was lost.

LOSSES AND SECRETS: SELF-HARM

For so many of these women the rage at their deprivation is manifested against themselves as they mutilate themselves in private, further damaging the points of contact between their own and other people's bodies. I have argued elsewhere (Motz 2001) that women use their bodies to articulate what cannot be spoken or thought about – that their bodies become quite literally the sites of battles and the modes of communication. It follows, therefore, that the most hidden and shameful secrets, like sexual abuse as victim or perpetrator, are likely to surface in memory with no verbal expression. That is, to describe or discuss these events is a potentially traumatic experience and the woman with severe personality disorder is more likely to attempt to escape from or encode this memory through action. One such action is self-harm, affording as it does a tremendous sense of relief and conversion of psychic to somatic pain.

Self-harm – only revealed as a fait accompli in blood, blisters and scars – is also a warding-off of contact. It seems at some level to be the creation of a false skin, warped and other, that keeps the woman apart from anyone who might try to touch her. The perverse aspect of self-harm, its narcissistic immersion, is also a powerful defence against intimacy. A concrete example of the hidden nature of self-harming is the discovery, in the X-rays taken after a women on the unit had broken her arm, of some 45 needles she had inserted into her skin, completely undetected by staff. Her apparently innocent, 'feminine' requests for the occupational therapist to help her develop skills in cross-stitch had this underlying motivation, with its deception, violence and perversion.

Self-harm can have a profound effect on staff, who are asked to witness these acts of violence and, to some extent, to take responsibility for them. The nurses in particular are asked to take on a maternal, protective role, tending to the self-inflicted wounds with kindness and concern. But these wounds are often shocking, repulsive and frightening to behold, conveying a sense of reproach and hostility: 'You didn't stop me from doing this – you allowed this to happen on your shift – look what I can make you do now.' Staff responses can be angry, in reaction to the unconscious communication of hostility by the self-harmer, and because of the sense of frustration, helplessness and despair that dealing with self-harm generates. It is a violent act, and can meet with a violent response. When staff become unable to think about the self-harm because they are too hurt, confused and assaulted by it, they may feel overwhelmed, out of control, and have a strong (shameful) wish to retaliate. This is clearly a potentially destructive situation, and one that demands reflection and working through.

I have described how some of the particular challenges and provocations unconsciously created by women with severe personality disorders are bound to invite retaliatory behaviour and feelings by staff, particularly those who work most closely with them. This is a dynamic that is painful to describe and even more painful to be caught up in, challenging as it does the staff's conceptions of themselves as carers – the feelings of wanting to care for and comfort that have been the conscious impetus for entering mental health care. Staff who choose to work in fields like mental health nursing may also have a powerful unconscious desire to be cared for themselves, which can lead to envy of the patients who receive this care (Menzies 1959). These feelings are very painful for staff to acknowledge and manage.

CASE EXAMPLE 2: CREATIVITY, RETALIATION AND ENVIOUS ATTACKS BY STAFF

In this setting it is very hard for the patients to retain the talents and modes of expression that were important aspects of their lives before the institution took over and further eroded their fragile sense of identity. It often comes as something of a surprise when women on such a ward exhibit their strengths, in singing, art, writing or other skills. It is as though the women have *become* their damage and disturbance, and their healthy, vital or creative aspects are totally located outside them in the talented staff. When the women's talents are exhibited, they are sometimes enviously and unconsciously attacked by the staff.

An example of this is the case of the missing poems and letters, which a very silent but articulate woman had been presenting to the nursing staff as gifts. Eventually it transpired that they had been thrown into the rubbish bin without being read, not even filed unread in her notes. Her communication was too painful and raw for the staff to bear. Being somewhat more removed, I found her writing beautiful (which was perhaps also a way of holding it at arm's length) and had gone looking for it. One letter, written in red ink, began 'Please consider this as written in blue, because today there is no blue pen.' Very personal and painful to read, it went on as a love letter, describing an early sexual encounter: 'I was excited as I thought no man would have me as I was brown…' She had discovered her letters in the bin, and confronted the housekeepers with the destruction of her work. She then took to her bed for over a week, refusing to communicate in any way. While her communication could not be heard by staff, she powerfully received their hostile response – she was witness to the apparent indifference and rejection to which her letters had been subject.

I want to end with this example, which shows how this woman's communication was collectively obliterated, to the great cost of her self-esteem and the possibility of therapeutic engagement. Returning to the theme of hiding and being lost, I want to make the final point that the hide-and-seek game, which has run as a theme throughout this chapter, has as its central aim the desire to be found. This to me is the key fact that we should bear in mind.

The hider who is never found is like the runaway whose absence is not noticed. I believe that the unconscious hope of these women is that they will, and can, be found by us; that they can make contact with us, and that we will find a way to bear their communication. The women's fear of, and desire for, closeness requires us to allow and encourage gradual steps towards therapeutic contact and a receptivity to the possibility of communication rather than a more persecutory approach. I believe it is through such an awareness and sensitivity to the central paradox for these patients that a genuine therapeutic engagement can be made.

10

Sharing Strength, Wisdom, Pain and Loss

A Women's Group in a Medium Secure Setting

Nikki Jeffcote, Tessa Watson,
Amanda Bragg and Sarah Devereux

INTRODUCTION

This chapter describes the first 21 months in the life of a women's group held on a medium secure ward for women. The four authors co-facilitated the group in three pairs during this period. We first describe the group's development, then discuss some of the themes of the group and its significance within the service as a whole.

BACKGROUND TO THE GROUP

Amberley Ward is a 17-bed women's ward within a large NHS secure service. The patients described in this chapter were a diverse group, ranging in age from late teens to mid-fifties. Two-thirds were single, just over half were mothers. Most had a history of disrupted care and sexual and/or physical abuse in childhood. Nearly half had never been employed. Many had significant physical health problems. Most had multiple diagnoses and their clinical presentations varied widely. All but one had a history of violence to others, and the majority had a history of self-harm and substance abuse. Just over half had convictions, ranging from minor acquisitive offences to major violence against the person. They had been admitted from the community, prison, open wards and other secure settings. Most were detained under civil sections of the Mental Health Act (1983), but nearly a fifth were subject to Home Office restriction orders.

ORIGINS OF THE WOMEN'S GROUP

The heterogeneity of the ward's 17 women, combined with the depth of disturbance, fear, anger and distress they experienced, presented both staff and patients with a huge challenge in attempting to create a therapeutic environment. Self-harm and assaults were frequent. Staff had difficulty balancing a predominantly medical, individualised model of care with the need to manage high levels of interpersonal conflict.

The need for 'crisis management', the women's diverse levels of functioning, and the lack of any therapy space on the ward contributed to great difficulties in establishing and maintaining group therapeutic activities. When the women's group started, the ward group programme consisted mainly of practical, time-limited activity groups. However, lessons had been learned from previous unsuccessful attempts to set up more reflective groups. Lack of trust between the women regarding disclosure of personal information, a perceived expectation to divulge that information, pressure on women to attend, and the lack of a defined group space had all contributed to the failure of previous psychotherapy groups.

The idea for the women's group came from our observation that the women had no space to talk about their experience as women. We were also aware that there was little consideration of womanhood in day-to-day clinical thought. For example, the emotional impact of physical changes caused by psychotropic medication (such as producing breast milk or periods ceasing) was rarely discussed. The loss of potential childbearing years was not acknowledged. Female experience and identity tended to be thought about in terms of pathology, for example, the possible role of pre-menstrual tension in increasing a woman's psychotic symptoms. The clinical team's structure and approach to the women was not noticeably different from the institution's traditional approach to its male patients. The size and disturbance of the ward disempowered women, who could only exercise control or choice by refusing to attend sessions or to co-operate with medical interventions.

The multiple demands of the ward made it hard for staff to find the time and space to reflect on their work, or to give stretches of undivided attention to individual patients. The environment was often inconsistent and unpredictable for the women; for example, escorted ground leave was frequently cancelled because of emergencies. The attempt to address the 'problem' of women patients by putting them together in one ward had to some extent replicated their previous invisibility. The aim of the women's group was therefore to acknowledge and articulate some of the important hidden realities of the women patients' lives and experience.

DEVELOPMENT OF THE GROUP

The setting

After negotiation with the ward staff and the women, it was agreed we would use a sitting room on the ward for the group. This room was to one side of the main ward and offered some protection from the noise and activity of the main day area. It had direct access to a secure balcony and there was a glass-walled smoking room in one corner.

We decided that drinking tea and coffee should be part of the group, as is usual in adult gatherings. On the ward, plastic cups and tepid water were used to reduce risk, but we negotiated with the team to use china cups in the group and to bring a kettle to boil water for the drinks.

We set a clear session length of 45 minutes and bought a small beanbag cat to use in an opening and closing 'round', marking the beginning and ending of the group sessions in a concrete but flexible way. The choice of the cat was serendipitous and, as described below, its anthropomorphic qualities gave it a special, symbolic value.

Group rules

We had three group rules:

1. Information shared in the group would be kept confidential unless the facilitators felt someone was at risk of harm.

2.   Everyone would participate as much as they were able to on the day.

3.   We would show respect for ourselves and each other in the group.

We chose these rules to try and establish an environment of reasonable safety in which every woman was entitled to a place, while recognising both the women's complex difficulties and the constantly changing environmental stresses they experienced.

Evolution in the early months

The group's structure evolved over the first few months. Taking time during the early weeks to find out what worked expressed the ethos of the group, in which the facilitators acknowledged they made mistakes, and getting something wrong did not mean it was a failure.

After having tea and coffee at the end, and then the middle, of the session, we found that drinking tea for 15 minutes at the start of the group worked best. The tea-making equipment was then put away, although the women could finish their drinks at their leisure, and the group meeting followed for 30 minutes.

Initially we used old, rather battered china mugs. However, it soon became clear how much the women valued being able to have a hot drink out of a china cup and we bought a set of mugs that became the group's own. Mugs could not be taken out of the sitting area, although they could be taken into the smoking room where the facilitators could keep track of them. The delicacy of balancing risk and responsibility in relation to the mugs is discussed more below.

In the early months of the group, the women would often regulate their participation by leaving to have a cigarette in the glass-partitioned smoking room. This seemed to be an important way of gaining some distance from the group while remaining in contact with it by sight. In the first summer, the women also started at times to use the balcony in a similar way. However, only part of the balcony was visible from the sitting area, so women could become cut off from the group. This occurred during a period of significant staff change on the ward, which had increased patients' insecurity and anger. Moving out to the balcony seemed to be a communication of anxiety and hostility. In order to contain this anxiety, we introduced a new rule that the balcony could not be used during the group. Despite some initial, rather uncertain, protests, the women accepted this.

In the first few weeks of the group's life we planned the sessions carefully and were fairly active in them. One week we introduced a 'family tree' exercise that did not work, being too challenging emotionally and cognitively. The following week we apologised for imposing, and then persisting with, the 'family tree' task. Acknowledging our mistake seemed to bring about a change in the group. The women began to talk to each other animatedly in a rising crescendo of sound, so all could speak and be partly heard, without having to take centre stage. From then on they took the lead in sessions, and over time spontaneously raised many powerful issues we had previously tried unsuccessfully to introduce in a more planned way. Only when a facilitator was leaving did we need to introduce more structure, to help the women deal with the anxiety raised by change and loss. However, the group's survival after the first departure of a facilitator marked an important strengthening of its confidence and safety. Over time, a sense of assurance developed that the group was owned by the women and could not be taken away by any individual leaving.

THE GROUP EXPERIENCE: THEMES AND ISSUES

In this section we describe some recurring themes and aspects of the group's life.

What it means to be a woman

We began the group with an idea of providing an opportunity for the women to talk about their experience as women. Some of the issues we anticipated would arise, concerning children, families, relationships, and the physical and emotional aspects of womanhood, did indeed recur throughout the group. However, the women found it hard to take these discussions very far because they were soon faced with the realities of their own lives, their lacks and losses, and with a sense that they had somehow put themselves beyond the community of 'ordinary women'.

Most women had some history of assaulting others, but there was very little talk of violence in the group. When it was discussed, it was usually in terms of being on the receiving end of violence from men. In one session,

Myra Hindley was discussed in the context of a news item that she was seriously ill but was not to be released from prison. The initial reaction was one of animation and anger at what was perceived as continuing victimisation. One of the more psychotic women then made a reference to the mother of one of the victims and her continued grieving, and the indignant discussion died away. It has been noted that staff working with women in secure services often have difficulty holding in mind the women's status as both victims and aggressors, and the women seemed to have the same difficulty.

Any mention of a husband or male friend tended to peter out quickly. There was occasional 'girls' talk', when the women spoke wryly and humorously about sex, differences in the way men and women approach the world, and relationships between people in the ward community. These moments created a sense of belonging, normality, sharing and identity but were hard to sustain. Conversations about children and motherhood were also difficult, and were usually approached from the position of being daughters and granddaughters rather than from being (or not being) mothers.

A distinctive characteristic was the group's rhythmic quality, its natural ebb and flow of energy, interest and focus. Sometimes the group was about sharing a cup of tea in a nice mug, at other times it was about expressing, communicating and sharing conflicts, losses, despair or happiness. There was no pressure to use the group in one of these ways rather than another, and no value judgement about one of these ways being 'better' than another. This seemed to contrast with the more 'masculine' dichotomies of progress and stagnation, success and failure, that underpinned most activities in the service.

The meaning of illness

The sense of something being 'not right' permeated the women's attempts to make sense of their situations. Every day they were surrounded by experiences of psychotic fragmentation, re-lived traumas, and actions that sought to change a state of mind or being that was felt to be unbearable. The fear of being mad was expressed in a range of different ways in the group. Some of the most psychotic women spoke of their fear of being dead, of being lost, of losing themselves. The less disturbed women often distinguished between themselves as 'normal' and the more disturbed women as 'insane'. Most seemed to experience a mixture of identification with women who were more troubled than they were on a particular day, and a sense of comfort and relief that they at least were not as bad as that. The women frequently showed great kindness and acceptance towards others who they could see experiencing greater torment, fragmentation and disorientation than they did.

Example: *Rosie, who is very ill, talks continuously. Maggie says agitatedly, 'Shut up, shut up, I can't bear it, I'll go mad'. Rosie says, 'I'm not a witch, am I?' Anna replies, 'No, you're a beautiful princess'.*

Overall, it was a characteristic of the group that every woman was able to 'hold court' at times, and that the women would attend to the sense and 'feel' of each other's communications, even when the actual speech was not quite intelligible.

Example: *During the opening 'round' with the cat, one of the women, Susan, talks at length in a mumbling psychotic way. The women listen respectfully and in silence. After a while Susan stops, looks up and studies the group, then says, laughing, 'Oh God, I'm talking rubbish!' The group laughs warmly with her. Susan, unusually, neither leaves the group nor becomes agitated.*

Sometimes women would use the group to 'leave' a statement about their state that day.

Example: *Rosie comes briefly into the group and when asked how she feels says, 'I feel like dying today'. She leaves soon after, distressed.*

The women rarely addressed the realities of being mentally ill in a direct way, but sometimes did so obliquely.

Example: *Most mugs were a bright colour with a picture of a fruit, but one showed a picture of a red-headed child with the words 'Ginger Nut' underneath. Over many months, this mug was rarely used, usually being the last to be chosen. Eventually, one of the women pointed out that it was 'not very nice' to have something labelled 'Ginger Nut'. The women then decided they did not want this mug to be brought to the group any more.*

Being a patient on Amberley Ward

What it meant in terms of power and vulnerability to be a patient and to 'belong' to Amberley Ward were themes addressed regularly, if sometimes indirectly, in the group.

The feelings of powerlessness and resentment provoked by compulsory medication, inconsistency in the environment and staff's failure to protect the women were often mentioned. Hope that the ward would help them take their lives forward alternated with despair that nothing ever seemed to change. Resentment at not being able to have a normal adult life alternated with a fear that such a life would not be manageable. Anger at the Amberley environment alternated with a fear that it would be even worse on the outside.

The difficulty of being an adult, and of 'acting one's age' in such an environment, was also discussed. The older women in particular felt alienated both from younger patients and from staff who were often many years their junior.

Example: *Maggie talks about feeling humiliated – as though she were aged five, at school. She mimics a member of staff waving a finger at her to tell her off. Then Maggie says how hard it is 'to think for yourself in an abnormal environment'. She talks of the difficulty of having a conversation with another person because the things you say 'bounce off the walls'. The only thing to do, two of the women agree, is be emotional. Maggie disagrees – you can't be emotional, distress is punished.*

The women also knew that other people were frightened of and did not want them. They were aware of the hospital culture that said 'It's awful working on Amberley' and of what this implied about themselves.

Exploring similarity and difference

Secure services tend to be structured to emphasise the differences between staff and patients. Hinshelwood (1987) discusses the way that:

> responsibility, together with the resources and power needed to meet it, comes to be relocated in the staff by common social agreement; and irresponsibility, together with the attendant sense of depletion and helplessness, accumulates in the patients. (p.16)

It was central to the atmosphere of the group as a community of women that we, the facilitators, were also women. However, as staff we had significantly more power than patients. We sought to acknowledge similarities without denying differences, and this was at times a difficult line to tread. We also tried to share responsibility for the group with the women from the start, and this was at times frightening for them and us.

Example: *At the beginning of the session, Maggie has the radio on very loudly in the smoking room. There is an unspoken awareness that if the facilitators intervene, the situation will escalate. Emma asks Kath to tell Maggie to turn the radio off, which she does. Maggie joins the group and says, 'Let's talk about African culture', then makes personal, abusive remarks to the two facilitators. Kath looks anxiously to the facilitators to manage the situation, Sara giggles nervously. Then Emma says, 'It's a good idea to talk about African culture' and shares some of her thoughts with the group. Other women join in. Maggie leans back dramatically in her chair and closes her eyes in a contemptuous gesture. Emma comments, 'She's gone to sleep' and continues to talk about her concerns about the ward. Maggie opens her eyes and listens quietly as others share their experiences.*

At times we also felt very anxious about how to manage disclosure of personal information. Many issues raised by the women were of concern to us too – issues to do with families, social and sexual relationships, children, our bodies, our self-image and our identities. It felt important to acknowledge this sameness, while protecting information that we did not wish to share.

Example: *The theme chosen by the women for discussion is 'Mothers and daughters'. The facilitators feel it is crucial to be able to answer personal questions in the right way. It would be easy to answer defensively or 'therapeutically' in order to avoid a difficult encounter. In the event, only a few comments are made towards us. It seems to be understood that nobody is expected to say anything if they do not want to, and that this extends to the therapists who can be accepted by patients as both women and therapists with professional boundaries at the same time. There may also be a fear among patients and therapists of the power of jealousy and envy in these profound areas of our lives.*

Change and lack of change

Amberley Ward experienced a much greater turnover of staff than of patients. While some staff departures were marked with a ward party, many were not and the women increasingly found a member of staff had just 'disappeared'.

Example: *There is discussion about staff leaving the ward. The women say they usually hear on the 'grapevine' about departures. Sometimes they hear on the day the person is leaving, sometimes after they have gone. Jo says this feels as though the person who has left is 'a non-person, someone who never existed'. Several women say it is better not to know in advance if someone is leaving. Sharon and Julie find this discussion too difficult and leave the group. Maggie says she is due to move to another hospital soon and would like a farewell party. Jo says she hopes to leave soon too, and Maggie suggests they could have a joint party. Jo is uncertain. At the very end of the session, Jo says 'Should old acquaintance be forgot for the sake of auld lang syne? – no, they shouldn't.'*

The departure of three of the facilitators allowed the women to show their awareness that staff seemed unable to stay long on Amberley, and to express guilt, anger, responsibility and fear about this. It was also important for the facilitators to share some of their feelings at going instead of pretending to collude with the idea that people were always glad to get away from Amberley.

Safety

A study of the women's perceptions of their own safety, carried out just after the start of the women's group, showed considerable fear of abuse, bullying and sexual harassment on the ward. It was therefore a priority to create a safe place in which to communicate and be with each other. We wanted to create a structure that supported the women without setting up other boundaries designed primarily to protect us, the facilitators. We sought to offer the women the highest level of freedom and personal responsibility compatible with acceptable risk.

Creating a safe and therapeutic environment meant taking risks. In the early weeks, we struggled between being too lax and too authoritarian. The 'participation' rule, which kept the group available to all the women while helping them take responsibility for how much they could tolerate, at first led, at times, to almost constant coming and going, which threatened the group's cohesion and safety. It took time for the group's timing, format and ground rules to act as the main 'container' for anxieties and conflict.

The china cups were also important in this respect. The women answered the trust the mugs represented by treating them responsibly. A woman once, in anger, flung a mug at a cupboard before walking out of the group. She did not aim or throw the mug anywhere near another group member, but this incident was a severe threat to the group and the women realised it. The woman who threw the mug was told she was still welcome in the group if she could abide by its rules, but she did not return for several months, as if she knew her action had been serious and threatening to the group. When she came back, she was able to moderate her anger in response to feedback about the importance of respect.

By taking risks ourselves in the group – with hot tea and china mugs, by tolerating verbal attacks, by not immediately intervening when there was conflict, and by being open to personal questions we were not sure how to answer – we seemed to enable the women also to take risks in terms of sharing information, relating in an open way to each other and taking responsibility for the safety and survival of the group.

The group's artefacts

The group acquired a range of objects, or artefacts, which fulfilled important functions in maintaining safety, consistency and continuity and embodying aspects of the group's experience.

The beanbag cat's anthropomorphic qualities allowed it to represent a 'member of the family' who could safely be loved, cared for, used as a weapon, hated and abused. Sometimes it was given a name, sometimes feelings were attributed to it, sometimes it was used as a mouthpiece. It could be taken care of by group members when they could not take care of themselves or each other.

At different times the women wrote their hopes and wishes on posters which, together with the group rules, were stuck on the wall at the start of each session. These were a reminder of continuity and the possibility of change, and were often used to facilitate new patients' membership of the group.

The kettle, mugs, drinks and biscuits symbolised the women's ability to have something they wanted and could enjoy. The teabags and biscuits were also sometimes a medium for expressing the feelings of isolation, privation and struggle for survival on the ward, as individual women tried to take several at once, or remove them from the group.

EVALUATING THE GROUP

We believe the women's group was – and is – a valuable part of the care offered to the women on Amberley Ward, but how do we know? We finish with a range of indicators that may be useful in making an objective assessment of the group's value.

Identification and discussion of important issues

Our session notes showed that the women were able to discuss issues they identified at the beginning of the group as being of concern to them. They also raised sensitive issues that we could not have introduced ourselves, such as rape and other sexual and physical abuse.

Attendance

Almost every woman on Amberley attended the group at some point. Some of the most disturbed and psychotic women were among the most regular attenders and could gradually stay for longer periods. For some, the women's group was the only therapeutic intervention they could manage.

Comparison with other women's groups

Most previous 'women's groups' had focused on self-care and grooming. They tended to fold after six or eight weeks. In this women's group, stereotyped feminine activities tended to be requested at times of high anxiety but once a sense of security was re-established, discussion re-focused on the losses, ambiguities and uncertainties of the women's lives.

Comparison with other Amberley groups

The women's group was (and is) by far the longest running therapeutic group on the ward. It was sustained partly because it could address staff departures without collapsing, and partly because responsibility for the group was shared between patients and therapists. The therapists did not 'carry' patients, and indeed experienced support and learning from them.

Disturbance in the group

The women's group was also characterised by a much lower level of disturbance than other groups. Sessions were never terminated prematurely and no woman was ever excluded from the group.

The women's views

Before writing this chapter, we discussed it with the women and asked them why they thought the group had lasted. They identified the following aspects of the group as positive:

- We look after each other.
- We exercise our minds.
- We acknowledge our differences.
- We can have an argument and make up.
- We discuss things women might do together.
- We appreciate one another.
- We talk about what's going on in our lives.
- We talk about the past.

Research with women

The group has engaged with several of the principles identified during development of the Government's national strategy for women, including:

- A focus on learning new behaviours, new coping strategies, new support structures, learning to take responsibility.
- A participative, user-led way of working.
- Creating a women's community.
- Providing containment, both physical and emotional.
- Consistency of care and relationships over a sustained and lengthy time period.

A Mental Health Forum of experienced women service users said they wanted therapists who:

- are women – if that is what we want
- listen
- treat us respectfully as individuals
- remember what we say
- help us make sense of what has happened to us
- genuinely care about us
- help us feel safe when we are talking to them
- help us feel safe after we have talked to them.

They also specified that they did not want therapists who:

- don't seem to care when we tell them about the awful things that have happened to us
- don't know how to help us when we want to talk about being abused and battered
- don't seem to know what to do if we get really angry or upset
- don't help us to keep ourselves safe
- patronise us and treat us like children
- don't treat what we say confidentially
- blame mothers. (Williams and Watson 1997, p.12)

We believe the Amberley women's group met many of these criteria.

CONCLUSION

In developing the group, we have not followed a specific theoretical orientation but have drawn on our wide range of cross-discipline knowledge and skills to develop a responsive, meaningful and therapeutic experience for the women. Not only we, the facilitators, but also the women patients in the group have had to take risks to achieve and use this experience, and we salute their courage.

NOTE

All names have been changed.

11

A Psychodynamically-orientated Group for Women with Learning Disabilities

Su Thrift and Carole Rowley

INTRODUCTION

This chapter is concerned with the first 24 sessions of a group that began in March 2002. After reviewing the literature we describe the women and their needs and go on to discuss important aspects of the group.

PSYCHOTHERAPEUTIC WORK WITH PEOPLE WITH LEARNING DISABILITIES

In an often-cited article, Bender (1993) noted that people with a learning disability were not generally offered psychotherapy despite a growing body of evidence as to the benefit of both individual therapy (Sinason 1992; Waitman and Conboy-Hill 1992) and group therapy (Hollins 1992; Szivos and Griffiths 1992). Reed (1997) noted that this client group has been one of the most ignored in terms of mental health services and psychological research into psychotherapeutic techniques.

National surveys suggest that this situation is changing and that clinicians are now offering a range of psychotherapies to people with learning disabilities. Nagel and Leiper (1999) attribute this shift to the wider transformation in societal attitudes. They state that it is no longer seen as appropriate to ascribe distress simply to a person's disability rather than to his or her emotional states and experiences. The concept that cognitive and emotional intelligence are distinct entities (Goleman 1998) has also been influential. Sinason comments that 'emotional intelligence may be left intact and rich regardless of how crippled performance intelligence was' (1992, p.6).

There is also a small but growing body of published literature that challenges the belief that people with learning disabilities cannot engage in or benefit from psychotherapy (Beail 1998; Berry 2003; Sinason 1992). However, as Arthur (2003) notes, whilst positive results of psychotherapy with people with learning disabilities are being reported, numbers of cases are small, there is still a lack of research in this area and it does not reach the level of sophistication achieved within the non-learning disabled population. There is only limited published literature on psychodynamically-orientated groups for people with learning disability (e.g. Gravestock and McGauley 1994; Jones and Bonnar 1996; O'Connor 2001). In thinking about our group we therefore drew heavily on literature about groups generally, and groups for survivors of abuse and those with a diagnosis of borderline personality disorder specifically (Campo-Redondo and Andrade 2000; De Zulueta and Mark 2000; Dickerson et al. 2000; Pines 1990). These papers gave clear descriptions and helped us to prepare for difficulties we might face, and to contain doubts about the group. Within this chapter we aim to give as honest an account as we can of the issues we encountered.

THE WOMEN AND THEIR NEEDS

The group meets weekly for 90 minutes with a ten minute break. It is comprised of two facilitators and four women who currently reside within the forensic service for people with learning disabilities at Brooklands, which is part of North Warwickshire Primary Care Trust. The women in this service are all assessed as having a learning disability. They have committed a variety of offences (including violent offences, fire-setting and sexual offences) and are detained on a range of sections of the Mental Health Act

(1983). Most have additional diagnoses including bipolar disorder, schizophrenia and recurrent depression. Many of the women have diagnoses of borderline personality disorder. Most have histories of severe, protracted physical, emotional and sexual abuse often by multiple perpetrators. Most of the women self-harm (including cutting, swallowing objects and inserting objects into their bodies) often to an extent or in ways that are life-threatening. They have been transferred to Brooklands from special hospitals, other psychiatric settings, and the criminal justice system.

These characteristics are similar to those of women in secure settings generally (Adshead 1994; Bland *et al.* 1999). Dorney (1999) notes that the shared experience of being a woman is rarely highlighted in the literature about people with learning disability. Readers may note similarities between the processes and issues raised in this group and those arising in groups for women without a learning disability who have similar histories and diagnoses. It is important, however, to maintain awareness of the women's learning disabilities and the effect of these on their lives. Many therapists view disability itself as a trauma (Hollins and Sinason 2000), involving loss of a 'normal self' and feelings of anger and shame about difference. People without learning disabilities may wish to avoid or deny the differences that come from disability because awareness of them arouses feelings of guilt and fear. It may also be difficult to face the depth and extent of loss that learning disabled people sometimes experience.

Many of the women's difficulties are connected to their early learning and abusive experiences. Some of their difficulties are also likely to have been exacerbated by their learning disabilities. People with a learning disability often have comprehension and communication difficulties and problems with recognising and labelling emotions. High intensity emotions such as those associated with experiences of early abuse, can be particularly confusing, difficult to express, and so are poorly managed or rejected (Gray *et al.* 1983; Reed and Clements 1989). Having a learning disability often involves difficulties with problem-solving, low self-esteem and poor self-efficacy. It may increase an individual's dependence on other people, leading at times to frustration, confusion, helplessness, anger, loss, shame and isolation. These feelings may be expressed in aggression to self and others, when they are usually labelled as 'challenging behaviours' within learning disability services. These behaviours have historically been managed using behavioural interventions that do not give people the opportunity to be actively involved in the process of change or to address wider issues about the causes of their distress.

THE GROUP EXPERIENCE

The group members expressed that their most pressing need was for a safe and containing place where they could talk about their overwhelming emotions. When they experienced such feelings in daily life the women often felt unable to contain these for themselves. They often believed they were not entitled to have needs, could not look after themselves and that others would not help them. As a result they tried to get their needs met, express themselves and relate to others in problematic ways. They repeatedly re-enacted well established abusive patterns in relationships with others. This led to further trauma and, at times, to violence towards self and others.

We will now look, in turn, at some of the main experiences of the group.

Emotional intensity

Given the women's histories and personality difficulties, it was inevitable that the emotions experienced within this group would be intense, extreme and labile, sometimes to levels that would be difficult to contain. These emotions were often linked to the women's past experiences of abuse. Terror and rage were common. Some of the women shook with fear in the group, and clearly felt exposed and vulnerable. They would hide their faces and blush, or say 'I wish you hadn't asked that.' They would also become angry and want to leave the room. They struggled with the desire to be known and understood and the fear of being seen as 'bad'.

Sometimes, issues related to events in the week would be brought to the group, particularly if one group member felt another had wronged her in some way. Hostility was expressed, usually in response to the perceived actions of the other person. These interactions often involved projective processes where the woman expressing the hostility saw something in the other that reminded her of a hated part of herself. For example, one woman said that another group member was bad because of her aggressive behaviour towards nursing staff. She took up a virtuous position which helped her feel good about herself despite her longstanding and recent history of violence to others. Anger arising from issues outside the group raised the challenge of how to keep the group separate from life on the unit where most of the women lived, whilst keeping it relevant.

One of the key roles of the facilitators was to bear strong emotion and to act as negotiators and mediators. The strength of emotion and powerful group processes at times led both facilitators to feel paralysed (unable to speak or move for short periods of time). We also felt clumsy about the words we used (although the other facilitator rarely agreed!), and had a sense of lost time. Such experiences may be linked to the helplessness and terror that are the sequelae of trauma generally. However, we also felt that the form these took was linked to the women's disabilities, particularly to the inability to communicate, and the fear of being 'stupid', 'dumb' and mis-understood.

Working with avoidance

It was often difficult for group members to stay with the intense emotion they experienced, and to deal with ruptures or conflicts in relationships in the group. They often avoided these issues, by moving on or suppressing their feelings. To manage this, when interactions became intense or confusing, one facilitator would continue with the ongoing interaction and discussion whilst the other attended to the group as a whole. This often resulted in an observation or reflection about the group that served to maintain cohesion and avoid fragmentation.

Although the women live together, they may manage emotion and conflict through avoidance. In their daily lives they may ignore each other or separate themselves by going to different parts of the building. Diffi-culties are often deflected or defused by nursing staff to prevent physical injury. As a result, the women do not necessarily explore or make changes to the way they interact with others, but repeat well-learned patterns that are often maladaptive. Within the group the women were encouraged to reflect on their feelings, thoughts and behaviour, and the consequences of these. Many of the women told of their difficulties when in previous groups. They had felt ashamed, isolated, unable to understand what was happening, and different from, or less able than, other group members. The women described how they struggled to be part of these groups, specifically relating this to issues of belonging and feeling welcomed. They had felt they were just tolerated, which caused pain and a desperate longing to be noticed and understood. However, they were also terrified about losing a sense of self when getting close to someone else, and had a desire to remain hidden. It is recognised that feelings of stigmatisation and not belonging are linked to abusive experiences (Finkelhor 1984), but issues of belonging may be particularly prominent for women with learning disabilities. They have often felt different from, and not as acceptable or valuable as, others within their own families or wider society. We repeatedly stated that all were welcome in the group regardless of their behaviour on the unit, and we noted that people were missed when they did not attend. The women described their fantasies that the group had forgotten them if they were not present for a short time, and their anger and sadness about this.

A number of strategies were put in place in an attempt to make it easier for the women both to attend the group, and to stay in the room physically, emotionally and cognitively. We tried to avoid repeating the women's negative experiences of other groups. First, the women were escorted to the group by nursing staff who stayed outside the room for the duration of the session. This ensured that if a woman could not tolerate staying in the room she could go outside for a short time and return later if she wished. Some group members would leave the group circle and sit in a different part of the room, returning when they felt able. It was made clear to the women that they were free to come and go as they needed. It was often a struggle for the women and the group facilitators to ensure that the women felt free to leave but also understood that they belonged in the group and were welcome.

Second, we provided art materials and puppets. We had originally envisaged these being used as an alternative means of communication, or to aid the understanding of concepts when using words was difficult. Initially, the women would draw frequently, and in later sessions would reach out for paper if they felt they could not communicate in words or were not being understood. The materials also enabled the women to externalise their feelings and thoughts without projecting them onto another person in the room, which allowed for a safe exploration of feelings. The women also drew pictures as a way of staying in the room without actively participating. We aimed to help the women to explore, at their own pace, emotions from which they would normally hide or flee.

Power

The women frequently discussed and enacted issues of power within relationships. They talked about situations when they felt they had power and control, and times when they felt out of control. They discussed situations when they knew they were trying either to gain or to lose power, and why and how they did this. In a number of sessions, group members expressed their anger overtly, shouting about how angry they were, raising a fist to another person, or slamming the door on their way out of the room. In other sessions the women talked about violent fantasies in which they were powerful and took the power away from others. One woman described imagining someone she perceived as frightening and threatening as a spider, whose legs she amputated until the spider was no longer able to move. Sometimes the women gained power through exaggeration of their disability, apparently becoming unable to understand an idea that they had previously understood. This appeared to link with Sinason's (1992) concept of secondary handicap. Here, the person is viewed as unconsciously exaggerating her or his actual disability as a defence against the anxiety and loss associated with the disability. This gives the person control by making the other feel 'stupid' instead. All these women have experienced powerlessness during multiple abusive experiences. Because of their learning disabilities they experience the powerlessness that results from not understanding when others can. In the group, the women explored sharing power rather than being either all-powerful or powerless.

At times it was a struggle for the group to contain these feelings. Expressing such feelings in violent ways had often contributed to the women's admission to forensic settings. Our attempts to keep the group safe, while allowing the expression of emotion, were not always successful and on two occasions one woman hit another.

A common experience for the facilitators was an awareness of their own power and the women's fear of this power, especially in the early stages of the group. We sometimes felt we were imposing our own agenda on the group. We felt intrusive when trying to encourage and support, and abandoning if we allowed space. We viewed this as a re-enactment of abusive dynamics.

People with learning disabilities do not always pick up on the subtle social cues or non-verbal communications that inform us about other people's emotional states or reactions to situations. They therefore may not understand how people infer thoughts and feelings. Therefore, when reflecting on a woman's emotional state it was vital for the facilitators to be explicit about the information on which they were basing their observation (e.g. tears, facial expression, body posture).

Unbearable need

Themes of envy (Klein 1997) were prominent in this group. Envy was expressed as a feeling of being deprived of something another woman had. Initially the women snarled at each other, sighed or tutted loudly and turned their backs on others who they perceived as getting something that they wanted for themselves. They interrupted, with statements that communicated it was 'their turn now', or that others were taking up too much space or being given too much. When they saw another group member seemingly getting their needs met, they wanted to spoil this. This usually took the form of a verbal attack, or an ostentatious, angry departure. In later groups, the women would verbalise such feelings. The women struggled to have enough space for themselves in the group, and were afraid that there was not enough care for everyone. They attempted to stay for extra time in the breaks or after groups. They requested individual time, or extra sessions with both facilitators. Each woman appeared to try and communicate that her problems were the most important or challenging, and that she needed more time and attention than the others.

REFLECTIONS ON A GROUP FRAMEWORK

We hope that we have demonstrated that running a group with women with traumatic histories, borderline personality disorders and learning disabilities is possible. These women were able to use the group to communicate their emotional experiences. In the life of the group so far we have felt both excited and confident about the group and its potential, and at times emotionally exhausted. We have had to find a range of ways to manage our experience, and the experiences of the group, and summarise these below.

Preparation

Before starting the group, we developed a written plan for the sessions. This helped us identify the need to be flexible and to adapt to the needs of the group. We gathered materials (including stories, games, puppets and drawing materials) for the women to use, as we were expecting that they would have some difficulty understanding or expressing concepts. We aimed to provide enough space for the women to be creative, and enough structure to prevent their misunderstanding, or becoming bored or anxious. We anticipated and discussed the potential for re-enacting abusive relationships (Dickerson *et al.* 2000).

We discussed the roles that we would expect to take and boundary issues that might arise. We anticipated that there would need to be a clear distinction for Carole between her roles as unit manager and group facilitator. We also had concerns that the women might feel coerced into attending because Carole was co-facilitating, and attempted to overcome this by having a consent process that was independent from the group facilitators.

We recognised the need to address the potential resistance to the group that we might face from others. Williams (1993) stresses the importance of organising the therapeutic system in order to work effectively. We had to work to contain anxieties in the wider system at various points during this group.

Supporting ourselves

We had a 45 minute planning period prior to each group session. We always met, but seemed to avoid planning the group, instead discussing other issues. Initially, we were concerned about this apparent avoidance, but we later came to see this as a time when we 'dumped' other concerns, making a space for the group. Initially we met briefly after the group before writing separate notes. However, this did not help us to process the emotion generated by the group and we began to feel isolated and split off from each other. We therefore decided to tape our conversations after the group to express and record our feelings. This helped us to maintain a real, coherent sense of the group without being overwhelmed.

We coped with doubts about the group's process and value, and our competence, by returning to the group literature and revisiting our aims for the group. We reminded ourselves that we were aiming for a 'good enough' group, not perfection.

Boundaries

We developed rules and boundaries about the number and frequency of sessions. There was a clear beginning and end to each group with a short relaxation tape. We drew boxes on a sheet that represented each week, and that were crossed through at the end of sessions. We were explicit about the things people could and could not do in sessions. This included not laughing at each other or talking over each other. The women interpreted these rules pictorially. We only ran the group when both facilitators were available, and informed the group of planned breaks well in advance. These boundaries were important in developing a sense of safety for the women and enabling them to know what would happen and when.

CONCLUSION

In describing our experience of the group we have not focused on or attempted to measure outcomes. Our main aim was to help the women overcome the great difficulties they had even being present in the group, before exploring issues of abuse and trauma. The main achievement to date is that all the women have maintained membership of the group, although attendance for some has been erratic. When asked, the women state that they want the group to continue and talk of their ongoing need for somewhere to feel safe enough to talk about their overwhelming emotions. The group continues to meet on a weekly basis.

Part III

Service Development

'FRAGGLES' is the name given to girls on 'hospital wings',
'Holloway shuffle' is the walk that medication brings.
Many of the women need special mental health care,
They're the ones that really shouldn't ever be placed there.
They're sick, they're ill, they need attention that prison cannot give
Many so depressed, confused, they lose the will to live.
Suicide attempts are made almost every day,
And sadly is achieved by some who see no other way.

From *Engraved with a Knife*
Wendy Cranmer
HMP Holloway

12

The Development of Medium Secure Services for Women

Tim Lambert and Maja Turcan

INTRODUCTION

Over the last ten years increasing attention has been given to the issue of women's care in psychiatric services, particularly with respect to secure provision. This chapter considers the initiatives, policies and research that have influenced the planning and provision of secure care for women during this time, and examines the clinical context of these developments.

POLICY BACKGROUND

Over the last decade, a number of reports and Government initiatives have focused on the need for mental health services to be, among other things, gender-appropriate and gender-sensitive. With regard to a forensic population, these have included the report of the Reed Committee (1992), the *National Service Framework for Mental Health* (Department of Health 1999), *Safety, Privacy and Dignity in Mental Health Units* (Department of Health 2000a), the NHS National Plan (Department of Health 2000b) and the National Strategy for Women (Department of Health 2002a).

The Reed Committee identified the risk of women's needs being over-looked in male-dominated environments. The Committee proposed positive action to counteract such problems and to ensure that women received care, treatment, accommodation and rehabilitation with proper attention to their personal dignity. The Committee's report particularly noted the disadvantage of black and other ethnic minority women, with a higher percentage of such women (than men) suffering from mental disorder and a higher proportion being on remand. The report also high-lighted the disproportionate numbers of women in high security due to limited options at lower levels of security, higher rates of drug-related admissions for women, and particular concerns regarding the lack of facili-ties for pregnant patients and for contact with children. The Committee's staff and training advisory group highlighted the need for gender awareness training and for a greater range of services for women.

In a Department of Health (1998a) press release, Baroness Jay emphasised the Government's wish to end mixed-sex accommodation in hospitals and suggested that 95% of services would achieve proper segrega-tion by 2002. However, few guidelines for secure women's services were then available (Kaye 1998). A later summary of current provision for women in medium secure services in the UK (Hassell and Bartlett 2001) pointed out that NHS medium secure services were predominantly mixed or male-only, and that single sex female wards were more likely to be found in the private sector.

THE NATIONAL STRATEGY FOR WOMEN

In October 2002, following a series of national consultation exercises, the document *Into the Mainstream* (Department of Health 2002a) was published. This drew together research and experiential information relevant to mental health services for women. The following characteristics were noted to be more common among women than among men in secure care:

- Transfer to secure care from other NHS facilities.
- A history of fire-setting and criminal damage (but violent and sexual offending were less frequent).
- A history of abuse and self-harm.

- Physical ill-health.

- Admission to secure services after behaviour for which no charge or conviction was made.

- Detention under a civil section of the Mental Health Act (1983).

- A diagnosis of personality disorder, especially of the borderline type.

- Being the minority group in terms of numbers – representing between 14% (in high security) and 16% (in medium security).

The document noted that very few women were likely to require 'Category B' security (a term derived from the prison system and now applied to high secure hospitals), and identified the need for easy transfer of women across levels of security.

Into the Mainstream also commented on the treatment options and conceptual frameworks relating to borderline personality disorder in women, and made several recommendations including the provision of 'adequate inpatient support'. Shortly after the *Mainstream* document was published, the Government released a guidance document, *Personality Disorder: No Longer a Diagnosis of Exclusion* (Department of Health 2002b), setting out guidelines for the development of services to personality-disordered individuals. This document proposed the creation of secure inpatient facilities for men with antisocial/dissocial personality disorder and made recommendations both for the development of care provision by general psychiatry services, and for the creation within forensic mental health services of identified teams to work with personality-disordered patients. However, while the document alluded to women with complex personality disorders, none of its recommendations was specific to women and there was no reference to the strategy for women as set out in *Into the Mainstream*.

Following development of the concept of 'dangerous severe personality disorder', a number of facilities in prisons and high secure hospitals are being created for men who are thought to represent this group, but the relevance of the concept to women is still not established.

In summary, there is still a lack of specialist services for women patients within the NHS, resulting in the inappropriate placement of many women both within existing services and in prison. Developments in secure services for women over the past decade have occurred largely within the independent or private sectors. Many NHS services continue to impose admission criteria that exclude many women with complex clinical needs, notably the presence of primary or substantial personality disorder and co-morbid substance misuse.

THE CLINICAL CONTEXT

There is now sufficient information available from official statistics and research to recognise certain clinical, historical and socio-demographic features that characterise the group of women for whom secure mental health facilities should properly be devised. This information has been drawn from surveys within women's prisons, Home Office statistics, and research carried out within high and medium secure mental health facilities. The clinical profile of women who may require secure care usually includes several of the following features:

- Co-morbidity of major mental illness, personality disorder, substance misuse, learning disability, educational disadvantage, post-traumatic symptomatology and/or psychosocial dysfunction.
- Serious or repeated offending.
- Disruptive, chaotic, assaultative, self-injurious or damaging behaviour.
- Significant physical morbidity.

There is little available research concerning women detained in general mental health services or in lower levels of security. However, it is recognised that women tend to enter secure services from general mental health units and to move up through levels of security, as well as entering secure care from the criminal justice system. It is not unusual for a woman to be admitted from an outpatient service to an acute inpatient setting and then, following escalation of behavioural disturbance and difficulties of management, to move through intensive care, low, medium and ultimately high secure care, very often without committing a serious offence or, alternatively, without any such offence reaching the courts. A question often raised part way through this process is whether the individual patient should be either discharged or referred to a higher level of security, and cogent arguments are often put forward for each course of action. A paradoxical situation may arise in which it is recognised that increasing the level of security may worsen the woman's behavioural disturbance and yet at each stage in the process the disturbance is such that no other course of action is seen as safe or acceptable.

RELEVANT RESEARCH

Ramsay et al. (2001) have described in broad terms some of the issues that relate to women and psychiatry generally and Kennedy (2001) argues for a proper focus on the needs of male patients. Both reinforce the need for gender-informed practice.

The literature now provides a fairly comprehensive description of key aspects of the clinical and offending profile of mentally disordered women who require secure care. Several important issues and themes have been identified by a number of authors as follows:

- mental illness, neurotic disorders and affective variant disorders[1,2,3,4]
- personality disorders[1,2,5,6]
- co-morbidity[2,3,6]
- substance misuse[1,4,5,6,7]
- abuse history[1,5,7,8]
- unmanageable behaviour[1,8]
- arson[2,5]
- serious violence, abnormal homicide[1,2,5,7]
- lack of education or skilled work, or a learning disability[5,7,8]
- previous time in a psychiatric facility or transfer from a psychiatric unit to a more secure unit (including high secure)[1,2,5]
- prison versus psychiatric disposal from court and use of Part II or Part III of the Mental Health Act[1,2,5,8]
- unmet treatment needs.[2,5,6,8]

1 Maden (1997)
2 Coid et al. (2000)
3 Rasmussen and Levander (1996)
4 Andersen et al. (1996)
5 Gorsuch (1998, 1999)
6 Lart et al. (1999)
7 Laishes (1997)
8 Maden et al. (1993)

Several other features are commonly encountered within this population. These include the emotional and behavioural impact of bringing together a number of patients who have high levels of co-morbidity, personality disorder and complex post-traumatic stress syndromes (Bercu 2001). Within a ward, there may be a wide age spectrum and a range of social and cultural sub-groups. Women with mild learning disability may share therapeutic resources with others of average or high intellectual ability. The wide variation in likely length of stay, from a few months to several years, implies different care and treatment needs, as does a spectrum of behavioural profiles from those who are well-organised, with high standards of self-care and interpersonal skills, to those whose behaviour is chaotic and unpredictable and may at times be provocative, challenging, intrusive, and offensive to others. Physical needs may also be highly variable, with fit women detained alongside older or more frail patients. Women with children, women without children, women who have been violent to or abducted children, women who have and have not experienced childhood abuse, may live together in a care setting but have widely different presentations and treatment requirements. The physical security needs of different women, and of an individual woman at different times, may encompass open or minimally secure settings, the spectrum of low and medium security, and more secure and intensive provision that enables de-escalation, containment of dangerous behaviour, and safe separation from others.

Aspects of the social environment are also relevant to the running of secure services for mentally disordered women. Important social and interpersonal phenomena include (Lambert 2001):

- the capacity for patients to act in concert with others or to become isolated

- the creation of gangs, cliques and scapegoats

- the emergence of a 'pecking order' and strong rivalries and jealousies

- the learning, mimicking and escalation of destructive, self-harming and assaultative behaviours, including absconsion, cutting, inserting objects, self-mutilation, arson and violence to others

- interference and intrusiveness, breaches of confidentiality and problematic sharing of information between patients, for example, concerning symptoms, treatment and personal history

- the impact of sexual behaviour that is disinhibited, abusive or predatory, or that heightens vulnerability to abuse

- drug use and trading

- the function of cigarettes as a medium for relationships and as a focus of conflict with staff and between patients

- the need at times to separate particular patients

- the impact of staff behaviour and dress

- managing contact and interactions with men, including male patients, friends, family and staff.

PRACTICES IN MEDIUM AND LOWER SECURITY SERVICES

Many NHS services are now revising their arrangements for women requiring secure provision. Research evidence and clinical experience indicate that in doing so, a number of key issues require attention:

- The need to create a sense of emotional safety and security.

- A physical environment that facilitates flexible care, management and treatment, including flexible arrangements for level and type of security.

- Adequate staffing levels, appropriate skill mix and the development of a culture of relational security, in which risk is managed and reduced through the development of supportive and containing relationships between patients and staff.

- The provision of adequate training, support and supervision of staff.

- Policies and procedures, including arrangements for procedural security, for example, searches, visits, access to lighters, responses to different kinds of boundary challenges, and use of leave and escorts.

- Family and attachment issues, including relationships with children.

- Improvement of mental and physical health, including the provision of 'well woman' clinics and dental, optician and chiropody services.

- Provision of a range of therapies.

- Provision of appropriate leisure activities.

- Educational and occupational opportunities.

Providing a service that can address these issues appropriately requires careful planning of the environment, staffing and patient groups. Defining clinical groups could facilitate the separation of those requiring high security from others and may also be helpful in determining the best way to match groupings of patients with location and treatment programmes. Coid *et al.* (2000) undertook a cluster analysis of 471 women admitted to high and medium secure services over a seven year period in the UK and commented on their security needs. Seven clusters were identified, each with a predominant diagnostic presentation but defined also by other characteristics such as offending and behavioural profiles. These clusters may be useful in guiding service development. One cluster, of women with primary antisocial personality disorder (who in many respects resemble a similar group of men in high security), was thought to include patients who might, in some cases, be likely to continue to require high secure services. Further research is needed to determine whether any of the women with a primary diagnosis of mental illness would require a high secure setting, as opposed to an environment with adequate relational and procedural security that focuses on the development of specific interventions aimed at managing and moderating 'treatment resistant' illnesses.

Clinical experience in existing dedicated secure services for women reinforces the importance of allowing adequate physical space and the capacity to separate individual patients and groups of patients. It is also increasingly recognised that individual patients may, on occasions or for periods of time, require treatment in a high-dependency environment. This may be for reasons as disparate as excessively challenging behaviour, pregnancy or physical illness. In the context of relatively small patient numbers, this presents a challenge in terms of design and cost. One approach is to create 'clusters' within larger wards, allowing two or more patient groups to be managed, with some separation, in an environment designed for between ten and fourteen patients. The nature and design of the physical space is thus as important as procedures and staffing arrangements in allowing management of interactions between individual patients and varying groups of patients and staff. Environmental design, technological advances and the creative use of flexible spaces and barriers are likely to be necessary to achieve a 'best fit' of resources, space and clinical requirements. A suggested method for cluster assignment within two broadly-defined populations of patients in secure settings has been described by Rice *et al.* (1990).

Conceptually, the environment will best support service needs if patients are accommodated in small groups within a ward, and are enabled to move relatively easily between different therapeutic or security settings. It should be possible to separate or reunite patients with their peers easily, and to allow controlled access to mixed-gender therapeutic, rehabilitative and recreational facilities. The organisational and staffing arrangements should afford continuity of relationships without impeding a woman's progress through her optimum pathway of care.

Medium and low secure inpatient services form only a part of a wider context of treatment environments and support networks. Formal links to, among others, general mental health services, community agencies, supported accommodation, outpatient services and prison healthcare are essential to minimise inappropriate placements and allow for the development of treatment models in a variety of settings.

THERAPEUTIC ISSUES

Medium secure units treating women patients as an identified group in single-sex provision, rather than as individuals in predominantly male wards, have, of necessity, developed an eclectic approach to therapeutic interventions. Medical treatments directed at symptom control are combined with psychological approaches that may extend beyond those generally found in mixed or male-only services. Physical treatments, largely pharmacological, have also required adaptation to reflect their particular impact on women with respect to side-effect profile, dosage and clinical context. Nursing and security procedures, such as the use of control and restraint techniques, also need to be applied in a gender-sensitive manner, for example, taking account of the potential for re-traumatisation of women with histories of physical and sexual abuse.

The choice and appropriateness of psychological treatments is influenced both by the personality difficulties these patients present with and by their other diagnoses. Forensic women patients in inpatient and outpatient settings commonly present with borderline personality disorder or borderline traits and (additionally) antisocial traits, as well as high rates of physical and sexual abuse (Turcan 2001). These characteristics reflect difficulties in trusting others and sustaining relationships and so have a significant impact on the capacity to engage with any treatment and to develop a therapeutic alliance.

The small number of forensic women patients, and their clinical and behavioural heterogeneity, makes systematic evaluation of specific treatment approaches highly problematic. Most forensic services for women therefore draw on treatments that have been evaluated with patients in general mental health services who present with complex difficulties. One such approach is dialectical behaviour therapy (DBT) (Linehan 1993). DBT is a broadly cognitive-behavioural approach specifically developed to treat borderline personality disorder in women. It was initially designed for an outpatient population but is increasingly being implemented in inpatient and forensic services. It offers a structured approach, involving both individual and group therapy, to help patients develop skills in self-regulation and effective management of relationships. Once a patient has gained control over damaging behaviours, such as self-harm or assaults on others, a more exploratory therapeutic approach, for example, psychodynamic psychotherapy or schema-focused therapy, may then be appropriate.

In terms of therapeutic techniques, DBT synthesises aspects of other approaches, including psychodynamic, cognitive, behavioural, humanistic and systemic orientations. Its strength lies partly in its coherent and integrated structure, which enables the emotional impact and intense interpersonal dynamics of work with highly disturbed patients to be addressed in a structured and explicitly problem-solving manner. In a review of treatments for personality-disordered patients, Bateman and Fonagy (2000) highlighted the importance of strong, coherent structures for therapeutic work with this group of individuals. They found that 'moderately effective' treatments tend:

- to be well structured
- to devote considerable effort to enhancing compliance

- to have a clear focus, whether that focus is a type of problem behaviour such as self-harm or an aspect of interpersonal relationship patterns

- to be theoretically highly coherent to both therapist and patient, sometimes deliberately omitting information incompatible with the theory

- to be relatively long term

- to encourage a powerful attachment relationship between therapist and patient, enabling the therapist to adopt a relatively active rather than a passive stance; and

- to be well-integrated with other services available to the patient.

These authors conclude by observing that the manner in which clinical treatment and protocols are structured and delivered is probably as important as the specific theoretically-driven intervention itself.

Despite the lack of formal evaluation, clinical experience suggests that such an approach, in which treatments are integrated and a shared 'ethos' maintained, may have promising results in terms of patients staying in treatment, reduction of damaging behaviours and the maintenance of effective teamworking among staff. Any attempt at a coherent approach of this kind requires that staff throughout the service have sufficient training to be clear about their roles and skills and to enable them to address problems and conflicts through shared concepts and terminology. A common language and understanding of the therapeutic model acts as a positive cohesive force within the service, diminishing the risk both of behavioural escalation within the treatment context and of staff burnout.

CONCLUSION

Over the past decade there has been a significant increase in knowledge about the clinical, offending and behavioural characteristics of women in secure mental health settings. It is now time to move from a focus on the commonalities among these women to a perspective that acknowledges their diverse needs and looks strategically at how the range of potential resources – in the community and in hospitals, in general mental health services and forensic services, in the NHS and in the private sector – can best be deployed. The challenge for the next decade is to develop and evaluate service provision and treatment interventions designed to meet the needs of those women who have historically found themselves in secure care.

13

Closing the Gap between Evidence and Practice

The Role of Training in Transforming Women's Services

Sara Scott and Jennie Williams

Gender and women's mental health cannot be mainstreamed in any sustainable way unless it becomes an integral element in the training of staff and managers at every level and within every organisation... In the longer term, these issues need to be incorporated into pre and post-graduate training for all mental health disciplines. (*Mainstreaming Gender and Women's Mental Health*. Implementation Guidance. Department of Health 2003, p.16)

What might secure services be like if all mental health staff were well-trained in social as well as biological and psychological perspectives and interventions? Almost certainly there would be fewer women than at present in secure hospitals and medium secure units. Community and acute services would be better able to work with the anger and distress underlying some of the relational difficulties – including aggression towards staff – that precipitate many women into secure services. For women living in these services there would be opportunities to form safe, therapeutic attachments to well-supervised staff; the institutional culture would be open and respect-ful, promoting mutual support; and patients would be regarded as adult partners working towards more socially and personally satisfying ways of living.

Unfortunately, nurses, psychologists and psychiatrists are still trained in traditions that barely acknowledge the social contexts of patients' lives and the psychological impacts of sexism, racism, poverty and abuse. Current training does not enable staff to provide empowering services that treat users as experts on their own lives and full partners in their recovery.

The necessity of addressing inequalities in mental health through changes in the training of staff has recently been recognised within the Department of Health by the Mental Health Care Group Workforce Team (MHCGWT) in conjunction with the National Institute for Mental Health in England (NIMHE) Workforce Programme. Work is underway to develop a core curriculum for pre-qualification training of all mental health workers which incorporates gender (and ethnicity) issues and attention to the specific needs of women. There are also indications that the national core competencies for mental health professionals will be redesigned to incorpo-rate gender issues/women's needs and there is a proposal for a national approach to developing staff training in issues of violence and abuse. Taken together these moves represent an unprecedented sensitisation of policy to the relevance of gender inequality in the provision of adequate health and social services.

Our intention here is to review how this change has come about, and to explore the steps that need to be taken to turn gender-sensitised policy ini-tiatives into the transformation of professional training. This chapter is therefore in two parts. The first briefly describes the building blocks for change as they have accumulated over the last decade. The second discusses some of the continuing barriers and the ways in which they may best be overcome.

THE STORY SO FAR

Until recently the integration of training to meet the strategic and clinical priorities of services has been patchy, to say the least. More recent policy (Department of Health 1998b) has recognised that if professionals are required to deliver a new mental health agenda then a much greater investment in training will be required. Specific skills have been identified in risk assessment and management, assertive outreach, home-based treatment and psychosocial interventions. Unfortunately, these interventions have been largely developed with the needs of, and risks posed by, male patients in mind; the relevant research and practice guidance in relation to these new treatment modalities is as gender *in*sensitive as has traditionally been the case. Indeed, the overwhelming majority of key mental health policy and practice documents make no mention of 'gender' or 'women' and consideration of any of the substantive issues relating to gender is extremely uncommon outside the Women's Mental Health Strategy (Department of Health 2002a).

An important exception is Standard 1 of the National Service Framework (NSF) for Mental Health which briefly acknowledges the inter-relationships that link gender, race, poverty, domestic violence and child abuse with mental health and social exclusion. It also attaches importance to identifying those 'key skills and competencies required throughout mental health services to ensure services which are non-discriminatory, and sensitive to the needs of all service users and carers regardless of age, gender, race, culture, religion, disability, or sexual orientation' (Department of Health 1999, p.21).

This overarching policy statement has been of immeasurable value to advocates and activists working to have issues of power and inequality recognised as core to providing appropriate services to people experiencing mental distress. During the development phase of the short course 'Working with Women in Secure Settings'[1] the fact that there was a wider policy context that at least paid lip service to these issues helped us to recruit pilot institutions. The NSF authorised issues of inequality to be brought out of the feminist and anti-racist margins and into the mainstream of service development.

---

1   This successful three-day course was the product of a partnership in 1998 between the University of Liverpool and WISH. Its development and piloting was led by Dr Sara Scott and funded by the Department of Health. Since 2002, Dr Jennie Williams at Inequality Agenda has been responsible for the development and provision of the course throughout the UK.

The Gender Training Initiative (GTI) – the project to develop training for staff working with women in secure settings – was set up in the same year the NSF was published and timing has in various ways been crucial to its success. In the late 1990s, Women in Secure Hospitals (WISH) was at the height of its visibility as a commentator on the inequity and inappropriateness of women's treatment in secure psychiatric services. As well as setting up the GTI to develop a tailored training intervention for staff working with women across the full range of secure environments, WISH commissioned two pieces of research. The first was an analysis of differences between men and women in the high security hospitals (Stafford 1999). This report describes the tendency for women's pathways to high security to include childhood abuse, disrupted care and education, little experience of paid employment, self-damaging behaviour, numerous psychiatric admissions, repeated assaults on staff or damage to property. Many women had arrived in high security because of the difficulties staff encountered in containing them in other psychiatric settings. These pathways contrasted sharply with those of many male patients who were much more likely to have committed serious crimes of a sexual and violent nature. This was the first time that gendered pathways into secure psychiatric services had been formally documented: such differences could no longer be dismissed as anecdotal.

The second piece of research commissioned by WISH was a consultation exercise on the views and experiences of women patients in high and medium secure units (Parry-Crooke 2000). This study found that the single most common source of women's dissatisfaction with staff was the lack of attention and understanding they received. The lack of respect and recognition women felt they were shown was experienced as grossly unjust: 'We are expected to behave like adults, but we are treated like children.'

Believing that the closer training could get to the everyday perspectives and difficulties of staff, the more likely it was to be able to encourage change, the GTI began with an assessment of training needs (Scott and Parry-Crooke 2001). From this it was apparent that many staff were perfectly aware of the inability of their services to meet women's mental health needs. Sixty multi-disciplinary members of staff across seven teams in six institutions (representing the range of secure provision in England and Wales) were asked to assess the relative importance for women's mental health of 15 different factors. It is evident from the findings shown in Table 13.1 that most staff identified the most significant causes of women's mental health problems as rooted in abuse and poverty, with least significance being accorded to genetic and biochemical factors.

Table 13.1 Rank order of the impact of different factors on women's mental health (N=60)			
Factor	Substantial or a lot	Some	None or a little
Emotional abuse in childhood	55	5	3
Low self-esteem	53	4	2
Childhood sexual abuse	50	6	2
Physical abuse in childhood	50	6	3
Poor problem-solving skills	46	10	4
Domestic violence	43	13	3
Disrupted early care	43	9	5
Hospitalisation/imprisonment	39	9	4
Gender roles	37	13	4
Poverty	34	17	3
Lack of educational opportunities	28	20	8
Lack of social networks	25	22	4
Racism	23	16	17
Biochemical factors	20	21	12
Genetic factors	13	15	23

These findings were confirmed in a study of mental health services provided by three NHS trusts and their partner agencies in the south of England (Williams and Waterhouse 2000). Almost three-quarters (72%) of the needs identified by staff could be regarded as gender specific, i.e. linked to women's gendered lives and experiences in their homes, communities and within mental health services. Findings also indicated that there was a clear recognition of the role of past and current abuse in determining women's mental health needs. However, the WISH patient consultation exercise suggested that from the patients' perspective there is a considerable gap between formal recognition of the issues in their lives and respectful, attentive and helpful responses from staff.

One of the impediments to change that was evident from the GTI research was that while staff recognised some of the social origins of women's mental distress and relational difficulties, they simultaneously held attitudes that stereotyped, disparaged and dismissed the women in their care. Women patients were frequently described as 'difficult', 'demanding', 'attention-seeking' and 'manipulative' and as 'more aggressive', 'less motivated' and 'more unpredictable' than men. Some descriptions offered in interview by staff of both genders revealed a barely disguised disparagement of women in general:

> [A]side from everything else, we have to work through menstrual cycles as well which is a nightmare. And of course females working on the unit have them as well. A group of women together. Ahh, evil! (Scott and Parry-Crooke 2001, p11)

Such comments suggest that the asymmetry of power between those who provide secure services and those who use services is also gendered and that it is intensified by gender inequality and misogyny in the wider society. One of the functions of such an accentuated 'us and them' situation is that it provides staff with a way of coping with their own feelings of hopelessness or incompetence. They can attribute the failure of women patients to thrive on the unit or ward to deficiencies in the women themselves rather than their environment; with anger, hostility and the desire to punish women being common emotional concomitants. These abusive group dynamics also provide staff with an inappropriate basis for group solidarity. At the same time it is demanding and risky for staff to listen properly to women patients (Lyon 1993). It means relinquishing stereotypes about their status and value, learning to communicate respectfully with each woman, and facing the very real possibility that they will have needs which staff have not been trained to meet.

LIMITATIONS IN TRAINING

Lack of relevant training, then, is one reason why services experience difficulties meeting the mental health needs of women. Findings from studies carried out over a number of years (Bolderston 1994; Williams and Watson

1991; Fernando *et al.* 1998) suggest that the training of mental health workers rarely enables them to use a social inequalities perspective. Few have had the opportunity to develop competence in linking social inequalities – including those based on sex, race, sexuality and age – to the mental health of individuals, or in using individual and collective approaches to empowerment. The GTI's training needs analysis of staff working with women in secure settings found that only a minority had received any training that had alerted them to the mental health implications of gender inequality. Only 15% reported that their initial training had addressed these issues. Few respondents had received any training about the effects of domestic and sexual violence on the lives of women and girls (20.6%) or on working with survivors of early trauma and abuse (26.9%). In the main, what training staff had been able to access had been optional and had taken place in the context of conference workshops.

It is not therefore surprising that while the majority of staff in the study by Scott and Parry-Crooke (2001) recognised that various forms of abuse had impacted on their patients' mental health, they were unclear precisely what the effects might be, what might be aggravating or mitigating factors, or how the 'problems in living' they observed had their origins in childhood relationships and traumas. The puzzlement of the staff nurse quoted below was typical of many responses to questions about the origins of patient's difficulties:

> I reckon a lot of the patients on our ward have been sexually abused when they were children [...and] that probably, to a certain extent, has contributed to the problems that they are having now. [... But] who knows? There are quite a lot of people out there that have been sexually and physically abused but got on with their lives and are living quite normal, happy family lives or career lives or whatever. (Scott 2000, p.8)

The GTI used this and other evidence collected through training needs assessments and semi-structured interviews to design a three-day course that would challenge gender stereotypes, encourage staff to take a more informed interest in both the origins of patients' difficulties and the role of services in their pathways to prisons and secure psychiatric services, and enable multi-disciplinary teams to take a new look at their work from a social inequalities perspective. During the past three years the course has served as a catalyst and adjunct to changes in the secure sector and over 40 courses have been delivered across the UK.

WORKING WITH WOMEN IN SECURE SETTINGS: COURSE CONTENT

The agenda for the course was set by the clear need to explore some of the realities of patients' lives in a way that increased staff confidence in engaging helpfully, and to provide opportunities for staff to re-frame some of the behaviour they find most problematic. Rather than locating its origins 'inside' the women – either in terms of their 'borderline' pathology or as a heightened version of 'what women are like' – we encourage the application of an inequalities perspective in relation to patients' past and present situations. In addition, we ask participants to consider issues of power and powerlessness as they exist between staff, and between staff and patients. It is the responsibility of the trainers to ensure a respectful, contributory workshop culture, in which no one is punished or humiliated for what they say or do, or for who they are. This includes male staff who are often in the minority, and who typically attend the courses with some trepidation. The intention is to create an environment where staff feel able to share concerns, try out ideas, draw upon personal experience, and think things through together. It should be added that this is a field where the participants' knowledge and expertise are not necessarily aligned with their status and position, so team members have new opportunities to feel valued and respected.

The course begins with a half day of group exercises designed to emphasise the cultural and historical variability of gender, and to disturb assumptions that contemporary gender differences spring 'naturally' from differences in genitalia and reproductive capacities. Recognising the potential and actual malleability of gender roles is a prerequisite for critical thinking about gender inequality. At the same time we introduce the idea that descriptions of gender issues are never neutral: that prior assumptions, frames of reference and 'investments' shape perception. Participants are also provided with opportunities to think about the ways that social inequalities shape society, and to focus on some of the ways that they have impacted on their own lives.

The course moves on to consider how assumptions about gender impact on ideas about mental health and influence assessment, diagnosis and treatment. Throughout the course we emphasise that gender difference is both material and ideological: thus women are the most frequent victims of sexual and domestic violence, but whether their accounts are listened to will be influenced by ideas about women being 'manipulative' and 'vindictive'. We invite staff to re-assess women's behaviours as the coping strategies of survivors, and to make sense of them in the light of the abusive relationships and disrupted attachments which characterised childhood and young womanhood for many of those in secure settings.

Research allows us to explore what is known about the different pathways to secure settings followed by men and women and the ways in which life experience and survival strategies interact with the views of judges, social workers and doctors (Carlen 1998; Stafford 1999; Allen 1987). Participants connect the generalised research portrait of 'women's pathways' with their own working experience by undertaking case studies of patients in their care.

The course embraces a paradigm shift: from a medical model that asks 'What is wrong with this woman?' to a social model which focuses on 'What has happened to this woman?' It follows a trajectory of very gradual change in UK mental health services over the last 30 years. Changes in professional training have not however kept pace with service developments. The course we have described here is an exception.

MISSED OPPORTUNITIES

At the same time as real momentum for change has been building, finding expression in the GTI and the recently launched Women's Mental Health Strategy (Department of Health 2002a), there have been some important opportunities to place social inequalities on the training agenda of mental health staff that have been missed entirely. One such was the United Kingdom Central Council's (UKCC) 'scoping' study on *Nursing in Secure Environments* (Storey and Dale 1999). In this document, discussion of the needs of staff working with women patients appears mostly under the heading 'Difficult Patients'. The unpopularity of working with women (and other 'difficult patients') is recognised, but the parts played by secure service culture, nurses' ignorance of the impacts of poverty, abuse and discrimination, and the misogyny of society in maintaining this situation are not acknowledged.

An opportunity to mainstream social inequalities into the core training of mental health workers was also missed by Lindley *et al.* (2001) in the first serious attempt to define the necessary capabilities of mental health workers. While their document, *The Capable Practitioner*, offers a promising formulation in a number of ways, it does not give clear direction about the place of social inequalities in its 'framework of capabilities'. So, while there is mention of 'managing diversity' and 'culture competence', words like 'abuse', 'power', 'powerlessness', 'inequality', 'discrimination' and 'oppression' are not part of the lexicon of this report. What is missing is any definition of the knowledge, skills and competencies needed to ensure that the mental health workforce is capable of responding constructively to the impact of social inequalities on the lives of service users. However, work is underway under the auspices of the MHCGWT to refine and develop this document (the 'Shared Capabilities Steering Group').

THE WAY AHEAD

A recent mapping exercise has explored the relevance of post-qualifying courses to supporting the implementation of the NSF for mental health (Brooker *et al.* 2002). Unfortunately, no attention was paid to the NSF's acknowledgement of the importance of social inequality to mental health and the necessity of non-discriminatory practice in the delivery of services. Instead, there was acknowledgement of wide regional differences in type and quantity of training, deficiencies in the knowledge of course tutors, insufficient service user input and a serious lack of multi-professional courses. The research team also identified that the rather few multi-disciplinary, skills-focused courses that did exist were attracting few 'psy'-professionals. The target intakes for psychologists and psychiatrists on relevant single module courses across the country were 4% (17 individuals) and 5% (20 individuals) respectively; in the previous year only one psychiatrist and no psychologists had been registered on these courses.

One interviewee in this study suggested that this could be changed if it were made a CPD requirement that 80% of CPD points had to be attained in a multi-disciplinary training context. This is the 'carrot' approach which may have to be supplemented by the 'rod' in some circumstances. Recognising the need for cross-disciplinary training, the GTI designed the 'Working with Women in Secure Settings' course to be delivered to multi-disciplinary, ward-based teams in the workplace – and the representative attendance of non-nursing staff forms part of the delivery contract.

In a discussion of barriers to learning, Horwath and Morrison (1999) suggest that staff working in secure contexts may show the highest resistance to training interventions:

> A group who share a very narrow view about practice, permit little discussion about difference and depend for their cohesion on mutual agreement will be very resistant to learning. Such groups can be encountered in most organisations, particularly in very closed settings, such as secure units. (Horwath and Morrison 1999, p.244)

If they are right – and our experience would confirm that in many secure contexts this is the case – then it is particularly important that training is taken into the workplace and is compulsory for all team members. However, this has implications for the selection of trainers who must be skilled at working with resistant, closed and ambivalent groups. For this reason the GTI resisted pressure to design an intervention based on a 'cascade' model. We believe that encouraging change based on a critical engagement with issues of social inequality requires considerable knowledge, experience (of the politics of organisational change and of interpersonal and professional dynamics) and skill.

There remains considerable difficulty in incorporating teaching on inequality into mental health training. There is no tradition of such teaching on which to build. The lack of 'clinically credible' staff in higher education is another factor and is likely to be of particular significance given that teaching in this area involves the presentation of perspectives that challenge the prevailing culture of nursing practice. A short-term solution may be to bring equalities 'champions', who are working and experienced in the field, into courses to teach appropriate modules. However, more robust solutions would involve the recruitment and training of specialist teaching staff.

GTI (now Inequality Agenda) trainers have been recruited throughout the country. Many work in secure services, others are service users who have been patients in the secure sector. All have participated in bespoke training delivered as an intensive residential course. A similar model could be used with clinically credible equalities trainers to deliver modules in higher education contexts. This might also help address Brooker et al.'s (2002) finding that user involvement in training often seemed superficial and tokenistic (they identified the MSc in Community Mental Health at the University of Birmingham as a notable exception). It is our belief that meaningful partnerships between professionals and service users are only possible where there is a real understanding of issues of power and inequality and a shared passion for far-reaching change (Williams and Lindley 1996).

SUPERVISION AND SUPPORT

The evaluation of the pilot 'Working with Women in Secure Settings' courses included an assessment of change at the levels of individual practice, ward culture and institutional arrangements six to nine months after training had been delivered. The extent of change was clearly related to a number of factors including the commitment or opposition of team leaders or consultants. However, follow-through of the issues raised by the course in the context of regular clinical supervision appeared to be the most important facilitating factor. This would seem to be confirmed by research on the impact of Psychosocial Intervention (PSI) training on routine service delivery. The existence of clinically competent local supervisors emerges as one of the key factors that make implementation of taught skills more likely (Brooker and Butterworth 1993; Milne et al. 2000).

The importance of supervision in linking training with practice cannot be overestimated. However, evidence suggests that supervision and support is a scarce resource across statutory mental health settings. Findings from the GTI's training needs analysis help to clarify what this can mean in practice. In this study staff were asked to state in which contexts issues of power and inequality were routinely addressed in relation to gender, race, poverty and sexuality. They reported that informal peer discussions provided the most common context for these discussions, and line management and clinical supervision the least common context. Many respondents (42%) in this study felt personally unsupported in their jobs, and even more stated that neither they nor their teams received adequate support or supervision to do their jobs properly.

Without a supervisory context in which reflection on both the interpersonal and social experience of patients and staff is authorised and facilitated, training intended to change practice will fail to do so. External supervision can bring fresh thinking into 'closed' environments and help open up pathways between secure, acute and community services for both service users and staff.

CONCLUSION

Validation, training and supervision of work from a social inequalities perspective will enable staff to close the gap between knowing what women want from mental health services and meeting their needs.

In terms of specific recommendations, we suggest there is a very strong case for national service standards around training and supervision for staff working with women in secure mental health services. It is crucial that the essential components of such training are clearly identified and we would endorse those laid out in the Implementation Guidance for the National Women's Mental Health Strategy (Department of Health 2003). This identifies the following as areas of competency that should be included in appropriate education and training:

- The social and economic context of women's and men's lives.

- Life experiences that may impact on their mental health, e.g. violence and abuse.

- The interplay between gender and other dimensions of inequality such as ethnicity, age and sexual orientation.

- Differences in the risk and protective factors for mental health in women and men.

- Differences in women and men in presentation and their pathways into services.

- Differences in the treatment needs and responses of women and men.

- The relationship between gender and power inequalities and how this may affect individual service users, staff and the organisations in which they work or are cared for.

- The day-to-day family, social and economic realities of women and men's lives.

14

Men, Women and Good Practice

Les Petrie and Nikki Jeffcote

GENERAL ISSUES

Introduction

The development of separate services for women has arisen partly from a recognition that gender is still an important dimension along which power differences fall. However, while the vulnerability of women patients is now acknowledged, the relevance of gender to staff, and to professional practice, has been less widely discussed.

In this chapter we first consider some of the general issues concerning staff gender in secure services for women. We then look more closely at aspects of practice that need attention in delivering a gender-aware service. We focus particularly on the contribution and support of male nursing staff, whose gender and close contact with patients produces particular pressures and demands. However, we want to emphasise that problematic practice and relationships are just as relevant to women staff, and that both male and female staff have a responsibility to be aware of the different kinds of challenge they each face.

There is virtually no literature on the impact and influence of staff gender on the day-to-day life of women's mental health services and those who work or live in them. The ideas in this chapter are therefore based on our clinical experience and observations, while also being grounded in the growing body of knowledge about women in forensic settings.

Male staff in women's services

On the whole, it is accepted that a mix of male and female staff is preferable in secure services for women. Women in Secure Hospitals (WISH), the main user and advocacy organisation for women in forensic mental health services, stresses the importance of positive male role models for women whose experience of men has typically been overtly or covertly abusive. Mixed gender staffing offers an opportunity for women patients to learn about the nature and boundaries of non-abusive behaviour, to build relationships with men that facilitate their own self-development, and to develop an awareness of the positive potential of differences between people.

Some services advocate an all-female staff team but in our view this is more problematic than helpful. It is an excessively limiting requirement when the pool of individuals who are motivated to work with women is often very small. It means excluding competent and empathic men. It conveys a message that men are always alien and untrustworthy, and that gender should have primary significance in how women negotiate their relationships. It risks conjuring a myth that only women are reliable caregivers. In a society where men still dominate positions of power, it also risks creating suspicion, jealousy and competitiveness that may lead to ghettoisation and, ultimately, marginalisation of women's needs and concerns.

To exclude male staff is to confuse male forensic patients with men in general. In ordinary life, women have some choice as to which male peers they associate with. Women patients do not have this opportunity. In mixed forensic services, women live with a group of men who are both unrepresentative of men in 'ordinary' life and, unfortunately, often rather more representative of the men the women have tended to encounter in their own lives. Most male patients in secure settings have been physically and/or sexually violent and, like the women themselves, often have very little experience of positive, respectful relationships. Male staff, by contrast, can offer women patients positive models of masculinity. The notion of role-modelling should be central to the philosophy of women's services and this includes the modelling of appropriate and respectful behaviour between the sexes.

It would also, in our view, be a mistake to think that services that are staffed only by women would be simpler or more 'problem-free' than those with mixed staff groups. Such a notion distracts from the very real issues facing female staff, whichever kind of staff group they are in. Inappropriate behaviour by women staff can be just as damaging as inappropriate behaviour by male staff. A focus on the sexual risks posed by the presence of men not only obscures the reality that women are also capable of sexual abuse, but also removes attention from other forms of inappropriate, harmful and anti-therapeutic behaviour. Identification between women can put pressure on boundaries in a number of ways. An atmosphere of 'sisterhood' may develop, blurring professional roles and obscuring the nature of the professional task. An example of this occurs when female staff and patients spend time grooming each other (e.g. plaiting each other's hair). Women staff may experience their sense of identification with patients as painful and frightening, leading them to behave in a punitive or rejecting manner. This may be particularly acute where there are dimensions of similarity in addition to gender, for example, shared social background or ethnicity. Envy and comparison are common and powerful features of many relationships between women and may be heightened in an all-female environment, just as the more overtly aggressive forms of competition between men tend to be exaggerated in all-male institutions. A mixed gender staff provides both sexes with a potentially creative balance, as well as reflecting social norms.

The dynamics of gender on women's wards

Patients, like staff, bring to their relationships assumptions about their own and others' behaviour as men and women. These assumptions are largely based on their personal experience and on the norms of their culture. Women patients have frequently suffered damaging and abusive relationships through much of their lives. They have developed expectations of others, and modes of coping and survival, that are associated with these experiences and arise from unmet needs for care and protection. The resultant dynamics affect both men and women staff.

Quasi-'parental' relationships are potentially problematic, particularly for staff who are motivated to work with women by a wish to provide reparative care. Such relationships reinforce the tendency to treat women patients as if they are children, and may become the focus for re-enactment of the women's original inadequate and abusive parenting relationships. Maternal attitudes and feelings can create unrealistic expectations of care and nurturance and arouse envy in other patients. Patients may have been let down severely by their own mothers, and often have at least as many unresolved issues around these maternal failures as around abuse by male caregivers. Younger female staff, particularly unqualified nursing staff, may represent a patient's 'successful' sibling, or the self she has not been allowed to become, again arousing envy that can lead, for example, to formal complaints and attacks on the staff member's professionalism. Staff who become pregnant may also create unbearable feelings of envy and hatred in women who have lost children or see little prospect of becoming mothers themselves.

Perceived and fantasised relationships with male staff can at times have a devastating intensity and reality, particularly for women who have been sexually and otherwise abused by men in their childhoods. Male staff are sometimes faced with highly sexualised behaviour, almost psychotic idealisation and hatred, and powerful pressures towards 'special' and intimate relationships. They are often unprepared for the complexity and intensity of emotions and expectations to which they are subject. The powerful relationship dynamics that emerge among groups of traumatised and disturbed women can also create pressures towards sexualised and aggressive behaviour between male and female staff, who may struggle to convey positive messages about male and female status and relationships.

It is important to acknowledge that sometimes staff are drawn to work in women's services for inappropriate reasons. Instances of workers applying to forensic women's services with the specific and deliberate intention of sexually targeting vulnerable patients are probably very rare (although the problems around such patients' testimony and credibility make them vulnerable indeed). But abuse occurs when staff act to meet their own needs in a way that overrides patients' needs, and this will not always be a conscious process. In our view, most instances of inappropriate behaviour that result in serious consequences are preventable. Such behaviour often develops gradually and can be addressed in its early stages. However, this requires a culture of openness and a readiness to monitor and challenge one's own and one's colleagues' behaviour.

PRACTICE ISSUES

Gender mix and task profile

As already noted, in our view forensic women's services should have a mixed gender staff group. WISH advocates a female:male staff ratio of 70:30, provided, of course that the male staff are able to work in a non-sexist way and realise that their behaviour as men is important. This ratio has also been endorsed by women patients and other representatives. However, from an operational point of view, a ratio of 80:20 is probably more realistic as there are a number of duties male staff should not perform. We believe these should include:

- Observations in patients' bedrooms.
- Observations in bathrooms.
- Observations in isolated areas.
- Administration of depot medication.
- Searching patients' bedrooms.
- Personal searches of patients on their return from leave.
- Supplying women with sanitary products.
- Intimate examinations.

Women should also at the very least have the option of a female primary nurse; in our view, primary nurses should always be female. Patients are encouraged to discuss their physical and sexual health, and other sensitive issues, within these relationships. The expectation that patients will talk openly about intimate issues is one of the ways in which the social rules of secure mental health settings differ significantly from the social rules of 'ordinary' life, and it is therefore particularly important to have clarity about the appropriate boundaries around this kind of disclosure and exploration.

Similarly, in our view no woman – whether she has been sexually abused or not – should be given a depot by a man or with a man present in the room. Ideally depots should never be given in a patient's bedroom; all services should have a separate treatment room for this and for all physical examinations.

Decisions about whether male staff should take women out on escorted leave need to be taken on an individualised basis, with a risk assessment carried out on each occasion. For both physical and psychological safety, male staff should stay in populated areas when escorting a patient. It is not appropriate to have a permanent, blanket 'no male escorts' rule for a woman. Risks consist of a range of factors that change and require regular review.

The different task profile of male staff can lead to playful or serious accusations by other staff that they are 'lazy'. Ironically, the male staff who are most aware of good practice – for example, refusing to take a woman's medicines to her bedroom – are often most vulnerable to this attitude. It is the responsibility of managers to ensure that male staff's qualities and contribution are appropriately used and valued by the whole team.

Managing behavioural disturbance

Many readers who work in secure women's services will at some time have been involved in, or witnessed, a woman's experience of distress, agitation and rage becoming so overwhelming that nursing staff feel they cannot manage the situation. They may then call for outside help.

From the perspective of the woman, what then happens is this: a response team consisting of four staff, often all men, rushes through the door towards her; the familiar objects around her are cleared away at high speed; she is physically grasped by these strangers, forced to the floor and held down by them in front of other staff and patients. Still in a state of acute fear and distress, she remains physically held while she is separated from the other women, her clothes are pulled down and she is given an injection in her buttock.

This is not an appropriate or helpful way to 'manage' a woman in crisis. It is traumatising, and frequently re-traumatising, for the woman, arousing feelings of intense fear, helplessness and shame. It is often also traumatising for the woman's peers and for staff who witness her terror and humiliation. It stimulates fear and anxiety in other patients (often perceived by staff as aggression or attention-seeking) that often leads to further assaults or self-harm. Other patients tend to feel a sense of identification and solidarity with the restrained woman and will not co-operate with staff.

We offer the following suggestions for good practice in such situations:

- Incidents should be managed by ward staff. As few staff as possible should be involved, and these should be women. If the response team is called, their role is to support ward staff, not to take over. Their presence on the ward is inflammatory and they should wait in a side room, to be available if they are needed by the ward team.

- The woman in crisis should be separated from other patients immediately and taken to a de-escalation suite. A de-escalation suite consists of a safe and calming room, with a lobby area, away from the main ward, equipped with safe furniture and soft furnishings. The door is never locked, staff are present at all times and they work to keep the patient orientated to what is happening. The aim should be to maintain contact and a relationship with the woman to enable her to work through the experience.

- The woman should be restrained 'sitting up', using a three-seater settee that enables staff to immobilise her while sitting next to her. This is consistent with views expressed by the Nursing and Midwifery Council and Royal College of Psychiatrists that 'pain compliance' techniques should no longer be considered acceptable.

Seclusion is not a helpful or effective way to manage psychotic or distressed episodes. It further isolates a woman who is already experiencing alienation from others. The impoverished environment of a seclusion room frequently reinforces the woman's urge to punish, which she may express in desperate actions such as stripping, banging her head and smearing faeces.

In situations where these guidelines cannot be followed, any male staff involved in a restraint need to be aware of the patient's anatomy and ensure they do not inadvertently touch her inappropriately, for example, on the breast. Male staff should never hold a female patient's legs during restraint as this represents the exercise of power over the lower part of her body.

Restraint is about technique, not strength, and trained female staff can manage incidents effectively. It should be possible to manage most incidents with no more than three staff. Assumptions that women are less competent than men in managing difficult situations should be challenged; it is important both for the service ethos and for patients' development that female staff are recognised as capable, effective and valued.

Complaints and allegations

Allegations by patients of inappropriate behaviour understandably create a great deal of anxiety among staff. The vulnerability of male staff to allegations of sexual assault by female patients is often informally quoted as one of the most 'scary' and off-putting aspects of working in a women's service. It is therefore important to highlight the following issues.

Allegations of inappropriate behaviour are made against both male and female staff. There is some evidence that in secure settings there is a greater risk of inappropriate sexual and sexualised behaviour by female staff towards male patients than by male staff towards female patients. In medium security, female staff receive as many, if not more, allegations of assault than male staff.

A view is occasionally put forward that allegations from female patients should be dealt with differently from allegations from male patients. This represents collusion with the idea that 'women lie' and is not justifiable. Policies for dealing with allegations must be consistent and consistently applied, regardless of the individuals involved.

Any allegation is traumatic for the staff member concerned. It is also potentially re-traumatising for the patient who has made the allegation and it will almost always have significant consequences for her, whatever the outcome. Each service's policy on allegations should require that investigations are dealt with quickly to minimise the stress to both parties. Investigators should be appointed equitably and should be given time out of their normal duties to complete the investigation. In these circumstances, most investigations could be completed in a few days.

Staff who are suspended as a result of an allegation should be supported by an independent counsellor and kept up to date regularly, for example by a weekly letter from the Human Resources Department.

If an allegation is found to be without substance, managers need to be aware that there will nevertheless be a legacy that requires acknowledgement and discussion. Support may be needed both for the staff member and the patient if they are to re-establish a therapeutic relationship. If resources permit, it may be appropriate to ask the woman if she would like to be transferred to another ward.

Preventing allegations

In a secure setting where staff and patients are in close proximity in an often highly-charged atmosphere, working with intensely emotional issues and a high level of disturbance, there will always be a risk of inappropriate behaviour. Maintaining clear and appropriate social, personal, emotional and physical boundaries is extremely challenging, and both staff and patients may come under strong internal and interpersonal pressure to breach them. Allegations, whether they have substance or not, always have a history and a pathway.

All members of the multi-disciplinary team therefore have a responsibility to support each other in maintaining appropriate behaviour and in monitoring any heightened risk of actual, perceived or alleged boundary-breaking. Breaches of ward rules and policies have to be addressed quickly and effectively. This involves not only ensuring that practice guidelines are adhered to, but also maintaining awareness in the team of why these guidelines are important. For example, a rule that a male staff member should not enter a woman's bedroom alone is important not just because it protects the staff member from allegations of unobserved behaviour, but also because a lone man entering a woman's bedroom may invoke for her a past relationship with a seductive or coercive abuser, and so set up a relationship dynamic that heightens the risk of untoward behaviour on one or both sides.

The whole team also need to monitor themselves and each other for increased attachment to, or involvement with, a patient. Staff may unwittingly make themselves vulnerable to misperceptions of their actions and to allegations. Physical contact may mean one thing to the staff member and quite another thing to the woman concerned. While a staff member may feel his or her 'special interest' in a patient is positive and therapeutic, the patient may (often correctly) feel that she is meeting a need of the member of staff, and may consciously or unconsciously seek to accommodate to this in ways that are damaging to both. Other patients may experience and act on feelings of jealousy and rivalry if they perceive any favouritism. Managers need to observe and be aware of attachments and behaviour that are not consistent with a safe, professional and therapeutic relationship, and should always address these with the staff member concerned. This is a role that, in our experience, managers often find difficult and awkward, and that they may therefore avoid. Training and supervision are needed to support managers in this aspect of their work.

Employing staff in women's services

Staff applying to work in a women's service need to know about some of the challenges that they will face, and services should ensure as far as possible that the staff they employ will respond appropriately when they are under pressure of various kinds. As part of the recruitment process, prospective staff should be given information about the kinds of difficulties the women have and how these may be manifest in the ward environment.

Ideally, staff should be recruited specifically to work with women and should have an expressed interest in doing so. Interviews need to explore issues of motivation and understanding of gender. Prospective recruits should also be given the opportunity to show that they can think about clinical issues in a non-sexist way and translate them into practice. Difficult situations should be outlined and the interviewee invited to comment on how these should be managed. This might well include a scenario concerning an allegation and suspension of a colleague.

When a job offer is made, references and qualifications must be checked, and an 'enhanced disclosure' protocol followed. Enhanced disclosure is operated by the Criminal Records Bureau (www.crb.gov.uk) and involves more thorough disclosure of convictions than is available through standard police checks. NHS trusts and other parent organisations must be prepared to take effective action to ensure that individuals who are known to exploit and abuse patients are not able to escape formal action or to leave quietly and get a job elsewhere. In the present employment environment this may take some courage and determination, and may cost money, but it is essential in stopping perpetuation of abuse.

Induction

New staff need an initial, competency-based introduction to working with women patients. This should cover the following:

- Patients' disclosure of sensitive information, including its appropriateness and ways of responding in a respectful, boundaried way.

- Dealing with sexualised conversations and inappropriate physical contact, including strategies to prevent these situations arising and skills for withdrawing from them if they do occur.

- Appropriate touch (no hugging, kissing, holding hands) and discussion of why this is important.

- Boundaries around personal information and ways of dealing with personal questions.

- The influence women's histories can have on how they perceive staff, and the way in which women's fantasies about staff may create pressure on the staff to step out of their professional role.

- The importance of role-modelling and the need to be aware of, and monitor, one's own behaviour with colleagues as well as with patients (to whom staff behaviour is highly visible).

- Presenting as a professional person, including consideration of appropriate and inappropriate clothing and the importance of not behaving in a sexual manner with either patients or staff on the ward.

These issues are relevant to all staff and should be revisited in ongoing supervision. We also suggest that male multi-disciplinary staff would benefit from their own meeting, perhaps twice a year, to share and discuss their particular experiences as men in a women's service.

Given that it is often difficult to recruit female staff, and in the light of a national shortage of trained nurses, it is essential to have an operational agreement that all agency/bank staff are inducted for the duties for which they are employed and that they have a general awareness of gender issues.

Training and supervision

There is a well established gender awareness training (see Chapter 13 of this book) that all staff in women's services should attend. This addresses issues of gender and other inequalities in society, highlighting their relevance both to staff and to patients. Education on trauma, its long-term effects and how it may be re-enacted is also essential in helping staff to understand the extreme emotions and behaviours they witness and work with. Theoretical and clinical knowledge also need to be integrated through training that combines reflection on actual clinical situations with role plays and videos that help staff to explore skills for dealing with them appropriately.

Supervision

All staff need individual supervision at which they can discuss personal clinical issues and their reactions and difficulties. It is important for supervisors to be aware of particular stresses and dynamics for staff of each gender. This supervision has to be separate from managerial supervision to facilitate open communication and confidentiality around private issues. However, supervisors also need to be confident and transparent about procedures in response to any disclosure by a staff member of unprofessional behaviour.

Multi-disciplinary group supervision that allows safe challenging of each other within a culture of professionalism is key to effective team functioning. Power hierarchies within teams can be paralysing but do not need to be; senior members of the team have a responsibility to make sure that junior and untrained staff are supported and enabled to participate fully. Group supervision should attend particularly to boundaries: between staff, between patients and between staff and patients. Procedural and relational boundaries are key to a safe environment and a team is strengthened by discussing these openly.

CONCLUSION

The current commitment to developing women's services within forensic mental health settings recognises the importance of gender in determining the way people behave towards each other. To build and maintain therapeutic environments for women patients, it is essential to pay attention to the particular skills and qualities contributed by both male and female staff. We hope that the ideas distilled from our experience and expressed in this chapter will support others in realising the therapeutic creativity that can result from informed, respectful and gender-aware practice.

15

A Gender-specific Advocacy Model, or 'I Found My Voice and I Love It!'

Laila Namdarkhan

INTRODUCTION

In this chapter I will discuss an advocacy model that is specific to women and tailored to the needs of women detained within secure mental health services and related environments. The model has grown from the experience of Women in Secure Hospitals (WISH) over the last 13 years, and it aims to be uncompromisingly women-centred and owned by those it serves.

I will begin by discussing the development of WISH over the past 13 years, with a commentary on the circumstances that have influenced its growth and work. I will then discuss the advocacy movement and WISH's advocacy model.

THE BEGINNINGS OF WISH

WISH began in 1990, inspired by women who were in the high secure system and by those who were leaving it. At this stage very little was known about this small but significant group of women. There was no recognition at that time that women in this situation needed a different type of security from men, or any awareness that women experiencing such high levels of distress required different care and treatment from male patients. There was a broad assumption that women could be 'tagged on' to the edges of services for men and that mixing both genders was therapeutically desirable.

It is now accepted in most quarters that women's presenting distress, then as now, largely has its origins in institutional, social and gender inequalities, prolonged violence, and sexual, emotional and physical abuse. To survive abuse, women develop complex coping strategies, such as self-harm, dissociation and somatisation, that have for the most part been seen as challenging and anti-feminine behaviours rather than a sophisticated lexicon of communications. In the early 1990s, women who presented in this way were at best seen as anomalous, at worst as highly dangerous. Once detained in the then secretive and closed 'special hospital' system, most women remained there for years, isolated, invisible and without any voice. Such women would later convey to WISH that these years had a catastrophic effect upon their ability to 'feel like a person'.

At this time, women lived in fear under degrading and humiliating regimes that in many instances dealt with them as wicked criminals rather than as women who required sensitive treatment for, and validation of, highly traumatised lives. Many were detained in conditions of higher physical security than necessary after being spiralled up the mental health system.

Blaming and punishing women for their own abuse and its consequences represents secondary abuse, which has often been perpetuated within the secure hospital system. We now know that women in secure hospitals have, over prolonged periods of time, experienced varying degrees of sexual harassment and actual assault by male patients. The system has sometimes responded to these situations with an expectation that women must tolerate such behaviour as preparation for living in the 'real world'. In other cases, extended inquiries have confirmed that women's stories are true and action has been taken to prevent further abuses. However, to WISH's knowledge women have never received public or private apologies for the system's failure to uphold their right to privacy, dignity and personal safety. There have also been few, if any, examples of perpetrators being prosecuted or seriously sanctioned, or of women taking a case to the civil or criminal courts for breach of duty of care. WISH believes this is further evidence of the secrecy and denial that surrounds abuse and violence within the system, affecting both women and men.

For many women who have experienced such secondary abuse, this situation leads to a further closing down of their world, where pain and self-blame are internalised. The process of becoming able to speak about these experiences requires consistent and valuing relational work by both staff and advocates. In many instances it can be years before women are able, if ever, to tell their stories and feel believed.

It was only in 1990 that WISH became one of the first independent organisations to be allowed into the high secure hospitals to gain access to women who were previously 'invisible' in the system. Advocacy of any sort was at that time a utopian ideal for both women and men detained in conditions of high security.

THE DEVELOPMENT OF WISH'S SERVICE TO WOMEN

There is no doubt that many professionals working in the system have been champions for a better deal for women and have worked with dedication to bring about changes that were by any standards hard to implement. But most would agree that women detained within the system first began to recount their stories, slowly and painfully, through WISH. In the 1990s and beyond, WISH's campaigning and relational work with women in secure hospitals had a significant impact on the way in which women's experience of the secure system was viewed.

During the past 13 years, WISH has been at the forefront of developments to put systems in place that provide what women need and want. Its frontline project work, which focuses on the development of consistent relationships, has provided a trusted, transparent and sustained conduit for the voices of detained women to be heard. WISH has developed long-term relationships with women, learning from them by listening without judging, by believing their stories, by working with them on an equal basis, reducing their isolation and letting it be seen, through regular visits, that they are valued as women who have the potential to move on in their lives.

Over this time, we have worked to try and achieve the provision of treatment and care that meet women's expressed individual needs in an environment that provides safe, positive relationships and non-obtrusive, non-oppressive security. It is now more generally understood that women patients need a gender-specific approach to their treatment and care and that heavy drug regimes, shock treatment, physical restraint and long periods in seclusion are counter-therapeutic. It is also increasingly recognised that harsh, rule-bound environments prevent many well-intentioned and empathetic staff from offering a humane approach to their patients. WISH believes that, if we are to move forward, professionals must engage with and own the reality of damaging past practices, however painful this may be. How the legacy of these practices is dealt with will be an important factor in ensuring that the changes women want and have campaigned for are actually achieved.

Throughout this period, the principal aim of WISH has been to work with women in ways that gain their trust, restore their confidence and, through long-term support, enable them to voice their views and concerns. We aim to offer a bridge of hope through participation in WISH.

RESEARCH

As well as giving a high priority to our frontline relational work, WISH has commissioned research to increase professionals' knowledge and awareness, inform strategy and so benefit women. *Defining Gender Issues* (Stafford 1999) made visible the gendered nature of the pathways that brought women into the system. This information contributed to the development of gender-specific training for staff working with women. The *Good Girls* report (WISH 2000) provided, for the first time, an account of what women said they wanted from the care system. Both documents have been used by service providers and commissioners to assist the development of new paradigms of care and treatment as well as informing the new mental health strategy for women, published in *Into the Mainstream* (Department of Health 2002a).

Since WISH began its work in 1990 there have been considerable changes within the culture of the NHS. It is now expected that the users of services should be involved in the planning and development of those services. WISH assumes that this is an inclusive model and includes women detained within secure mental health forensic services. We hope that our advocacy model will assist women in continuing to increase their participation and influence, both in their current situation and in the wider arena of their future lives.

THE ADVOCACY MOVEMENT

The concept of advocacy is not new. It has existed for many years in the fields of learning disability, mental health and the disability rights movements and there is a national advocacy network. This model offers empowerment to those who have historically been disempowered in many aspects of their lives by discrimination based purely on their 'difference'. The advocacy movement has involved people speaking up for themselves and demanding the right to access and enjoy the same privileges and services as the majority of the population. This has been achieved with the support of others, or by supporters speaking up on behalf of the disempowered group. Collective 'speakouts' and public demonstrations have drawn attention to social inequalities and blatantly discriminatory practices, while one-to-one advocacy has enabled people to articulate more specific issues concerning access to resources.

Within secure mental health services advocacy was slow to materialise. It began to emerge in the early 1990s in response to recommendations by public inquiries at the three high secure hospitals. Despite initial resistance, by the mid-nineties formal advocacy was implemented in two sites, although it did not arrive at the third site until 2001 and there was no liaison or sharing of experience between the hospitals. In all three cases, a generic, gender-neutral model was adopted, although Ashworth subsequently sought tenders for a gender-specific advocacy service. Women advocates were available as part of the service provision for women patients, but advocates worked across the gender spectrum, with an underlying expectation that a gender-neutral service would be offered.

WISH would certainly not argue that an advocacy team comprised of both women and men workers cannot deliver a gender-sensitive service to women. However, we believe that to do this it must be informed by an understanding that delivering advocacy to women requires a discrete, stand-alone service and not one that is bolted onto a generic gender-neutral provision. Only in this way can advocacy for women be protected from the pressures recognised by the Reed Committee (1993) which stated that: 'In male-dominated environments, women's needs...are liable to be overlooked.' The report also identified 'the need for positive action to counteract these problems and generally to ensure that women receive the care, treatment, accommodation and rehabilitation they need with proper attention to their personal dignity' (p.41).

DEVELOPING THE WISH ADVOCACY MODEL

WISH continued to provide its well-developed gender-specific relational service to women on all three sites alongside the new advocacy services, supporting workers where appropriate and ensuring that confidential boundaries between the work of WISH and the advocates were observed.

However, during a review undertaken in 1999, WISH's three Branch teams, for London South, the Midlands and the Northwest, began to look at developing a formal advocacy process based upon WISH's existing work. After considerable consultation and discussion, we came to the conclusion that WISH had in fact been using advocacy in its work, but it was a form of advocacy that was specifically informed and regulated by the needs of the women who engaged with us. The essence of our work was its emphasis upon building open, equitable and non-judgemental relationships with women, and its focus on process, rather than on issues and outcomes.

In many respects this represented the opposite of the established advocacy services. WISH was providing a fully independent service, funded separately from the locations in which it operated. Its frontline workers were engaged with women in an independent relationship that was not focused on their medical history, treatment or clinical outcomes, since these issues are expressed in a perspective and language that frequently pathologises and disempowers them. WISH manages these relationships in partnership with the women, within well-maintained and fully explained boundaries. WISH workers have learned that the ability to relate information transparently is crucial to the health and sustainability of these relationships, and they incorporate a pragmatism that recognises that women have to manage their lives on a daily basis (both in and out of services) under conditions that are fraught with constraints and frustrations. Surviving the system requires a great deal of energy and detracts from women's ability to concentrate on their own issues and to consider options that are safe and valuing for them.

The new national strategy document, *Into the Mainstream*, highlights the importance of the following issues in the development of services for women:

- Recognition that gender inequality significantly contributes to women's mental ill-health.

- The importance of listening effectively and respectfully to women and validating their experiences.

- The need for all mental health services to develop a gender-sensitive approach.
- The need for gender-specific services, of which some should, in accordance with women's wishes, be women-only.

These principles suggest that a review of current advocacy models in existing services – whether NHS, independent, mixed-gender or women-only – is appropriate, together with the development of gender-specific advocacy services. Women in secure mental health settings have experienced social exclusion and disempowerment over protracted periods, including their time in hospital, and this has rendered them silent over many years. For most, their wishes and personal boundaries have been ignored or destroyed from a young age and their only means of communication have been physical – graphically marked on their bodies in self-harm, manifesting in physical 'complaints', or expressed through violent actions that reflect the destruction of their own body boundaries and the trauma of past 'caring' relationships. Complex dissociative coping strategies create inner worlds that allow women to feel safe and secure from the traumatic reality of their experiences but also create intense social isolation. To access women who have endured such experiences requires a process that acknowledges the reality and validity of this experience and offers a space that allows for the building of trusted relationships. WISH's gender-sensitive advocacy model can support the breaking-down of these barriers and complement the long-term work that dedicated care teams are striving to achieve.

KEY FEATURES OF WISH'S CURRENT MODEL

The key features of WISH's current model are drawn from our experience of providing a gender-specific advocacy service at Ashworth Hospital for 12 months from 2002. This has been based on the following three principles.

Self-advocacy

It could be argued that including self-advocacy in our model is not exactly groundbreaking. Self-advocacy is traditionally concerned with speaking up for yourself and making your concerns and wishes clear to those who have some measure of agency over your life and your ability to act independently.

WISH fully endorses this aim and works with women towards self-advocacy and the raising of their own voices.

However, we also recognise that, for all the reasons already indicated, some women may not be able (or may choose not) to advocate for themselves. Because of the women's historical disempowerment, self-advocacy may not be immediately achievable. Using a range of approaches flexibly, while also striving with the women in open partnership towards using their own voices for themselves, is therefore essential. It has been our experience – endorsed by the women – that listening to and validating women's concerns and experience in the context of a gradually developing relationship, without imposing clinical or other interpretations, allows each woman to have control of the process and to make her own decisions about if, when and how to progress her issues. Within this process each woman has at all times the choice to self-advocate, to self-advocate with support, to have the advocate speak for her or to take no action. When she does wish to take action, she can explore a range of options, outcomes and relevant information with the advocate, and has the opportunity to rehearse interactions with professionals. WISH believe that only by giving a woman control over this process can she be empowered to grow over time towards true self-advocacy.

The focus of WISH's model on process rather than issues and outcomes does not mean that such a service is not accountable to those responsible for its commissioning. On the contrary, all services delivered by WISH operate within the terms of a detailed service agreement and are subject to quality monitoring and regulation, with regular customer satisfaction analysis.

Relational security

It should now be clear to the reader that WISH's relational philosophy is central to its model for a gender-sensitive advocacy service. This philosophy includes the belief that constructive, non-judgemental and confidential relationships are essential in helping women to feel safe, and in enabling them to achieve a sense of security that can protect them, and others, from actions born of overwhelming fear and distress. Intrinsic to this is the ability to work sensitively and with clarity to the women's agenda at a pace that suits her needs.

A second aspect of WISH's relational focus is its work with those who deliver services to women. This aims to support staff in developing their own relational capacities through training and dialogue, by acknowledging that their job is not easy and by helping them to understand both the women's situation and the wider system. WISH is concerned to build healthy and respectful partnerships that facilitate communication with staff and between staff and their women patients.

Being pro-active

WISH's monitoring and evaluation of its current service delivery has shown that being pro-active, in other words, actively making contact rather than waiting for women to ask for an advocate, has resulted in a very high level of advocacy contact with women. As a result, very few issues have needed to be dealt with reactively. Over the past year, only 3% of all contacts between women and WISH advocates were noted as reactive.

Being pro-active involves a high level of informal interaction and relationship-building with women alongside any specific advocacy that is needed. This is achieved through regular weekly visits in which relationships grow. Confidence in these relationships enables women to make good use of the advocacy service. They do not need to agonise over whether or not to make initial contact, and can prepare with advocates for significant reviews about their care in good time.

CONCLUSION

In summary, WISH believes it has developed a model of advocacy that takes into account the diverse abilities and situations of this small but important group of women. The model's overall goal is to support and encourage women to self-advocate; women themselves have ultimate control over how their views are advocated.

WISH recognises that we are at a developmental stage of providing advocacy services to women. However, monitoring and feedback so far indicate that the service model has been well received both by commissioners and, perhaps more importantly, by women who are actively using it with varying degrees of confidence. WISH has always opened its services to external scrutiny and would welcome the opportunity to participate in an evaluation of its advocacy model. In its current form the model aims to meet the needs of women detained in secure forensic mental health services, but we believe it can also benefit women who use general mental health services. Failing to listen to women and take their views into consideration is a mistake that new services surely cannot afford to make. WISH has demonstrated through its work that it is possible to listen and respond to women and to develop a service that is informed by what they have had to tell us. We hope that over time many more women will feel empowered to speak for themselves through being involved with WISH and through further development of WISH's model of advocacy for women.

Acknowledgements

The author would like to thank both past and current members of staff at WISH for enabling her to write this chapter and to all the women out there who are so generous with their support.

References

Adshead, G. (1994) 'Damage: trauma and violence in a sample of women referred to a forensic service'. *Behavioural Sciences and the Law 12*, 235–249.

Adshead, G. (1998) 'Psychiatric staff as attachment figures'. *British Journal of Psychiatry 172*, 64–69.

Adshead, G. and Morris, F. (1995) 'Another time, another place'. *Health Service Journal*, 9 February, 24–26.

Allen, H. (1987) *Justice Unbalanced; Gender, Psychiatry and Judicial Decisions*. Milton Keynes: Open University Press.

Andersen, H.S., Sestoft, D., Lillebaek, T., Gabrielsen, G. and Kramp, P. (1996) 'Prevalence of ICD 10 psychiatric morbidity in random samples of prisoners on remand'. *International Journal of Law and Psychiatry 19*, 1, 61–74.

Arthur, A. (2003) 'The emotional lives of people with learning disability'. *British Journal of Learning Disabilities 31*, 25–30.

Atkinson, L. (2003) 'Not a suitable place for girls'. *Howard League Magazine 21*, 19.

Bateman, A. and Fonagy, P. (2000) 'Effectiveness of psychotherapeutic treatment of personality disorder'. *British Journal of Psychiatry 177*, 138 143.

Baunach, P.J. (1985) *Mothers in Prison*. New Brunswick, NJ: Transaction Books.

Beail, N. (1998) 'Psychoanalytic psychotherapy with men with intellectual disabilities: a preliminary outcome study'. *British Journal of Medical Psychology 71*, 1–11.

Bender, M. (1993) 'The unoffered chair: the history of therapeutic disdain towards people with a learning disability'. *Clinical Psychology Forum 54*, 7–12.

Bercu, S. (2001) 'Experience of a women's psychiatric ward in London'. *XXVI International Congress on Law and Mental Health*. Abstract. Canada: Cheneliere/McGraw-Hill.

Berry, P. (2003) 'Psychodynamic therapy and intellectual disabilities: dealing with challenging behaviour'. *International Journal of Disability, Development and Education 50*, 1, 39–51.

Bion, W. (1959) 'Attacks on linking'. *International Journal of Psychoanalysis 40*, 308–315.

Bland, J., Mezey, G. and Dolan, B. (1999) 'Special women, special needs: a descriptive study of female special hospital patients'. *The Journal of Forensic Psychiatry 10*, 1, 34–45.

Bolderston, H. (1994) 'What they don't teach you on clinical psychology training courses'. *Feminism and Psychology 4*, 2, 293–297.

Bowlby, J. (1951) 'The making and breaking of affectional bonds'. *British Journal of Psychiatry 130*, 201–10 and 421–31.

Brooker, C. and Butterworth, C. (1993) 'Training in psychosocial intervention: the impact on the role of the community psychiatric nurse'. *Journal of Advanced Nursing 18*, 583–590.

Brooker, C., Gournay, K., O'Halloran, P., Bailey, D. and Saul, C. (2002) 'Mapping training to support the implementation of the National Service Framework for mental health'. *Journal of Mental Health 11*, 1, 103–116.

Cadden, J. (1993) *Meanings of Sex Difference in the Middle Ages.* Cambridge: Cambridge University Press.

Campo-Redondo, M. and Andrade, J. (2000) 'Group psychotherapy and borderline personality disorder'. *Psychodynamic Counselling 6*, 1, 17–30.

Carlen, P. (1983) *Women's Imprisonment.* London: Routledge and Kegan Paul.

Carlen, P. (1998) *Sledgehammer: Women's Imprisonment at the Millennium.* London: Macmillan.

Casement, P. (1985) *On Learning from the Patient.* London: Routledge.

Cavadino, M. and Dignan, J. (1997) *The Penal System.* London: Sage Publications.

Chipchase, H. and Liebling, H. (1996) 'Case file information from women patients at Ashworth Hospital: an explanatory study'. *Issues in Criminological and Legal Psychology 25*, 17–23.

Coid, J., Kahtan, N., Gault, S. and Jarman, B. (2000) 'Women admitted to secure forensic psychiatry services'. *Journal of Forensic Psychiatry 11*, 2, 275–295.

Cox, M. (1996) 'Psychodynamics and the special hospital: "Road blocks and thought blocks"'. In C. Cordess and M. Cox (eds) *Forensic Psychotherapy: Crime, Psychodynamics and the Offender Patient. Part 2 Mainly Practice.* London: Jessica Kingsley Publishers.

Davies, R. (1996) 'The inter-disciplinary network and the internal world of the offender'. In C. Cordess and M. Cox (eds) *Forensic Psychotherapy: Crime, Psychodynamics And The Offender Patient. Part 2 Mainly Practice.* London: Jessica Kingsley Publishers.

Dell, S., Robertson, G., James, K. and Grounds, A. (1993) 'Remands and psychiatric assessments in Holloway Prison'. *British Journal of Psychiatry 163*, 634–644.

de Zulueta, F. (1993) *From Pain To Violence: The Traumatic Roots Of Destructiveness.* London: Whurr.

de Zulueta, F. and Mark, P. (2000) 'Attachment and contained splitting: a combined approach of group and individual therapy to the treatment of patients suffering from borderline personality disorder'. *Group Analysis 33*, 4, 486–500.

Department of Health (1998a) *End in Sight for Mixed Sex Accommodation in Hospitals.* Press Release. London: DOH.

Department of Health (1998b) *Modernising Mental Health Services: Safe Sound and Supportive.* London: HMSO.

Department of Health (1999) *National Service Framework for Mental Health.* London: HMSO.

Department of Health (2000a) *Safety, Privacy and Dignity in Mental Health Units.* London: HMSO.

Department of Health (2000b) *The NHS Plan. A Plan for Investment, a Plan for Reform.* London: HMSO.

Department of Health (2002a) *Women's Mental Health: Into the Mainstream. Strategic Development of Mental Health Care for Women.* London: HMSO.

Department of Health (2002b) *Personality Disorder: No Longer a Diagnosis of Exclusion.* London: HMSO.

Department of Health (2003) *Mainstreaming Gender and Women's Mental Health.* Implementation Guidance. London: DoH.

Dickerson, J., Porter, J. and Jellema, A. (2000) 'Child sexual abuse survivors group: selection, group process and supervision'. *Clinical Psychology Forum 135,* 31–34.

Dolan, B., and Bland, J. (1996) 'Who are the women in special hospitals?' In C. Hemingway (ed) *The Experience of Women in the Special Hospital System.* Aldershot: Avebury.

Dorney, M. (1999) 'Group work with women with learning disabilities'. *British Journal of Learning Disabilities 27,* 132–136.

Edwards, S.M. (1984) *Women on Trial.* Manchester: Manchester University Press.

Fernando, S., Ndegwa, D. and Wilson, M. (1998) *Forensic Psychiatry, Race and Culture.* London: Routledge.

Finklehor, D. (1984) *Child Sexual Abuse: New Theory and Research.* New York: Free Press.

Fonagy, P., Target, M., Steele, M., Steele, H., Leigh, T., Levinson, A. and Kennedy, R. (1997) 'Morality, disruptive behaviour, borderline personality disorder, crime, and their relationships to security of attachment'. In L. Atkinson and K.J. Zucker (eds) *Attachment And Psychopathology.* New York: Guilford Press.

Gilligan, C. (1982) *In a Different Voice: Psychological Theory and Women's Development.* Massachusetts: Harvard University Press.

Gilligan, J. (1999) *Violence: Reflections on our Deadliest Epidemic.* London: Jessica Kingsley Publishers.

Goldson, B. (2003) 'No more excuses: a reasoned case for abolishing child imprisonment'. *Howard League Magazine 21,* 5–6.

Goleman, D. (1998) *Working with Emotional Intelligence.* New York: Basic Books.

Goodman, J., Salyers, M., Mueser, K., Rosenberg, S., Swartz, M., Essock, S., Osher, F., Butterfield, M. and Swanson, J. (2001) 'Recent victimization in women and men with severe mental illness: prevalence and correlates.' *Journal of Traumatic Stress 14,* 615-645.

Gorsuch, N. (1998) 'Unmet need among disturbed female offenders'. *Journal of Forensic Psychiatry 9*, 3, 556–570.

Gorsuch, N. (1999) 'Disturbed female offenders: helping the "untreatable"'. *Journal of Forensic Psychiatry 10*, 1, 98–118.

Gravestock, S. and McGauley, G. (1994) 'Connecting confusions with painful realities: group analytic psychotherapy for adults with learning disabilities'. *Psychoanalytic Psychotherapy 8*, 2, 153–167.

Gray, J.M., Fraser,W.L. and Leudar, I. (1983) 'Recognition of emotion from facial expression in mental handicap'. *British Journal of Psychiatry 142*, 566–571.

Hannah-Moffat, K. and Shaw, M. (2000) 'Thinking about cognitive skills? Think again!' *Criminal Justice Matters 39*. London: Centre for Crime and Justice Matters.

Hare, R. D. (1991) *Manual for the Psychopathy Checklist – Revised.* Canada: Multi-Health Systems.

Harris, G.T., Rice, M.E. and Quinsey, V.L. (1993) 'Violent recidivism of mentally disordered offenders: the development of a statistical prediction instrument'. *Criminal Justice and Behaviour 20*, 315–335.

Harris, M. (1998) *Trauma Recovery and Empowerment: A Clinician's Guide for Working with Women in Groups.* New York: The Free Press.

Hart, S.D. (1998) 'Psychopathy and risk for violence'. In D. Cooke, A.E. Forth and R.D. Hare (eds) *Psychopathy: Theory, Research and Implications for Society.* The Netherlands: Kluwer.

Hassell, Y. and Bartlett, A. (2001) 'The changing climate for women patients in medium secure psychiatric units'. *Psychiatric Bulletin 25*, 340–342.

Heads, T., Taylor, P. and Leese, M. (1997) 'Childhood experiences of patients with schizophrenia and a history of violence: a special hospital sample.' *Criminal Behaviour and Mental Health 7*, 117-130.

Heaven, O. (2000) 'The special needs of foreign nationals in UK women's prisons'. In R. Horn and S. Warner (eds) *Positive Directions for Women in Secure Environments.* Leicester: The British Psychological Society.

Hedderman, C. and Gelsthorpe, L. (1997) *Understanding the Sentencing of Women.* Home Office Research Study 170. London: Home Office.

Heidensohn, F. (1996) *Women and Crime.* London: McMillan.

Heney, J. and Kristiansen, C.M. (1997) 'An analysis of the impact of prison on women survivors of childhood sexual abuse'. *Women and Therapy 20*, 4, 29–44.

Her Majesty's Inspectorate of Prisons for England and Wales (1997) *Women in Prison: A Thematic Review by HM Chief Inspector of Prisons.* London: Home Office.

Her Majesty's Inspectorate of Prisons for England and Wales (2001) *Report on an Unannounced Follow-up Inspection of HMP Holloway.* London: Home Office.

Her Majesty's Inspectorate of Prisons for England and Wales (2003) *Teenagers in Prison Report.* London: Home Office.

Hinshelwood, R.D. (1987) *What Happens in Groups: Psychoanalysis, the Individual and the Community.* London: Free Association Books.

Hinshelwood, R.D. (1994) *Clinical Klein.* London: Free Association Books.

Hinshelwood, R.D. and Skogstad, W. (2000) 'The dynamics of health care institutions'. In R.D. Hinshelwood and W. Skogstad (eds) *Observing Institutions: Anxiety, Defence And Culture In Health Care.* London: Routledge.

Hollins, S. (1992) 'Group analytic therapy for people with a mental handicap'. In A. Waitman and S. Conboy-Hill (eds) *Psychotherapy and Mental Handicap.* London: Sage Publications.

Hollins, S. and Sinason, V. (2000) 'Psychotherapy, learning disabilities and trauma: new perspectives'. *British Journal of Psychiatry 176,* 37–41.

Home Office (2001a) *The Halliday Report (Making Punishment Work: Review of the Sentencing Framework for England and Wales).* London: Home Office.

Home Office (2001b) *The Government's Strategy for Women Offenders.* London: Home Office.

Home Office (2002a) *Statistics on Women and the Criminal Justice System.* London: Home Office.

Home Office (2002b) *Criminal Statistics England and Wales.* London: HMSO.

Horwarth, J. and Morrison, T. (1999) *Effective Staff Training in Social Care: From Theory to Practice.* London: Routledge.

Houck, K.D.F. and Loper, A.B. (2002) 'The relationship of parenting stress to adjustment among mothers in prison'. *American Journal of Orthopsychiatry 72,* 4, 548–558.

Hough, M. (2003) *The Decision to Imprison: Sentencing and the Prison Population.* London: Prison Reform Trust.

Hudson, B. (2002) 'Gender issues in penal policy and penal theory'. In P. Carlen (ed) *Women and Punishment: The Struggle for Justice.* Culhampton: Willan.

Jones, A.M. and Bonnar, S. (1996) 'Group psychotherapy for learning disabled adults'. *British Journal of Learning Disabilities 24,* 2, 65–69.

Kaye, C. (1998) 'Hallmarks of a secure psychiatric service for women'. *Psychiatric Bulletin 22,* 137–139.

Kennedy, H. (2001) 'Do men need special services?' *Advances in Psychiatric Treatment 7,* 2, 93–99.

Klein, M. (1997) *Envy and Gratitude and Other Works 1946–1963.* London: Vintage.

Laishes, J. (1997) *Mental Health Strategy for Women Offenders.* Canada: Correctional Service.

Lambert, T. (2001) 'Development of a secure women's ward from a group of mixed gender services'. *XXVI International Congress on Law and Mental Health.* Abstract. Canada: Cheneliere/McGraw-Hill.

Langan, N.P. and Pelissier, B.M.M. (2001) 'Gender differences among prisoners in drug treatment'. *Journal of Substance Abuse 13,* 3, 291–301.

Lart, R., Payne, S., Beumont, B., MacDonald, G. and Mistry, T. (1999) *Women and Secure Psychiatric Services: A Literature Review.* Report to the NHS Centre for Reviews and Dissemination. York: University of York NHS Centre for Reviews and Dissemination.

Liebling, A. (1992) *Suicide in Prison.* London: Routledge.

Lindley, P., O'Halloran, P. and Juriansz, D. (2001) *The Capable Practitioner.* London: Sainsbury Centre for Mental Health.

Linehan, M.M. (1993) *Cognitive Behavioural Treatment of Borderline Personality Disorder.* London: The Guildford Press.

Lloyd, A. (1995) *Doubly Deviant, Doubly Damned: Society's Treatment of Violent Women.* London: Penguin.

Luntz, B. and Widom, C. (1994) 'Antisocial personality disorder in abused and neglected children grown up'. *American Journal of Psychiatry 151,* 670–674.

Lyon, E. (1993) 'Hospital staff reactions to accounts by survivors of childhood abuse'. *American Journal of Orthopsychiatry 63,* 3, 410–416.

Maden, A. (1995) *Women, Prisons and Psychiatry.* Oxford: Butterworth-Heinemann.

Maden, A. (1997) 'Are women different?' *International Review of Psychiatry 9,* 243–248.

Maden, A., Curle, C., Burrows, S. and Gunn, J. (1995) *Treatment and Security Needs of Special Hospital Patients.* London: Whurr.

Maden, A., Curle, C., Meux, C., Burrow, S. and Gunn, J. (1993) 'The treatment and security needs of patients in special hospitals'. *Criminal Behaviour and Mental Health 3,* 4, 290–306.

Maden, A., Swinton, M. and Gunn, J. (1994) 'Psychiatric disorder in women serving a prison sentence'. *British Journal of Psychiatry 164,* 44–54.

Maden, A., Taylor, P., Brooke, D. and Gunn, J. (1996) *A Survey of Mental Disorder in Remand Prisoners.* London: Home Office.

Mental Health Media (2002) *What Women Want.* Videotape. London: Mental Health Media.

Menzies, I. (1959) 'The functioning of social systems as a defence against anxiety'. In I. Menzies Lyth (1988) *Containing Anxiety in Institutions. Selected Essays Volume I.* London: Free Association Books.

Mezey, G. and Bartlett, A. (1996) 'An exploration of gender issues in forensic psychiatry'. In C. Hemingway (ed) *Special Women? The Experience of Women in the Special Hospital System.* Aldershot: Avebury.

Milligan, R.J., Waller, G. and Andrews, B. (2002) 'Eating disturbances in female prisoners: the role of anger'. *Eating Behaviors 3,* 2, 123–132.

Milne, A. and Williams, J. (2003) *Women in Transition – A Literature Review of the Mental Health Risks Facing Women in Mid-life.* London: Pennell Initiative for Women's Health.

Milne, D., Keegan, D., Westerman, C. and Dudley, M. (2000) 'Comprehensive outcome evaluation of brief staff training in psychosocial interventions for severe mental illness'. *Journal of Behaviour Therapy and Experimental Psychiatry 31*, 87–101.

Monahan, J., Steadman, H.J., Silver, E., Appelbaum, P.S., Robbins, P.C., Mulvey, E.P., Roth, L.H., Grosso, T. and Banks, S. (1999) *Rethinking Risk Assessment. The MacArthur Study of Mental Disorder and Violence*. Oxford: Oxford University Press.

Motz, A. (2001) *The Psychology of Female Violence: Crimes Against the Body*. London: Brunner Routledge.

Nagel, B. and Leiper, R. (1999) 'A national survey of psychotherapy with people with learning disabilities'. *Clinical Psychology Forum 129*, 14–18.

Newburn, T. and Stanko, E. (1994) *Just Boys Doing Business? Men, Masculinities and Crime*. London: Routledge.

Notman, M.T. (1991) 'Gender development'. In M.T. Notman and C. Nadelson (eds) *Women and Men: New Perspectives on Gender Differences*. London: American Psychiatric Press.

O'Connor, H. (2001) 'Will we grow out of it? A psychotherapy group for people with learning disabilities'. *Psychodynamic Counselling 7*, 3, 297–314.

Parkes, T. (1997) 'Reflections from the outside in: my journey into, through and beyond psychiatric nursing'. In S. Tilley (ed) *The Mental Health Nurse – Views of Practice and Education*. Oxford: Blackwell Science.

Parry-Crooke, G. (2000) *Good Girls: Surviving the Secure System*. London: WISH.

Peay, J. (1997) 'Mental health and crime'. In M. Maguire, R. Morgan and R. Reiner (eds) *The Oxford Handbook of Criminology*. Oxford: Clarendon Press.

Penfold, P.S. and Walker, G.A. (1984) *Women and the Psychiatric Paradox*. Milton Keynes: Open University Press.

Perkins, R. and Repper, J. (1998) 'Different but normal: language, labels and professional mental health practice'. *Mental Health Care 2*, 3, 90–93.

Pescosolido, B.A., Gardner, C.B. and Lubell, K.M. (1998) 'How people get into mental health services: stories of choice, coercion and "muddling through" from "first-timers"'. *Social Science and Medicine 46*, 2, 275–286.

Pines, M. (1990) 'Group psychoanalytic psychotherapy and the borderline patient'. In B. Roth, W. Stone and H. Kibel (eds) *The Difficult Patient in a Group: Group Psychotherapy with Borderline and Narcissistic Disorders*. Monograph 6, Madison: American Group Psychotherapy Association Monograph Series.

Prison Reform Trust (2003) *Troubled Inside: Responding to the Mental Health Needs of Children and Young People in Prison*. London: Prison Reform Trust.

Quinsey, V., Harris, G., Rice, M. and Cormier, C. (1998) *Violent Offenders: Appraising and Managing Risk*. Washington DC: American Psychological Association.

Ramsay, R., Welch, C. and Youard, E. (2001) 'Needs of women patients with mental illness'. *Advances in Psychiatric Treatment 7*, 2, 85–92.

Rasmussen, K. and Levander, S. (1996) 'Symptoms and personality characteristics of patients in a maximum security psychiatric unit'. *International Journal of Law and Psychiatry 19*, 1, 27–38.

Reed, J. (1992) *Review of Health and Social Services for Mentally Disordered Offenders and Others Requiring Similar Services.* Final Summary Report. London: HMSO.

Reed, J. (1993) *Review of Health and Social Services for Mentally Disordered Offenders and Others Requiring Similar Services. Volume 5: Special Issues and Differing Needs.* HMSO: London.

Reed. J. (1997) 'Understanding and assessing depression in people with learning disabilities: a cognitive-behavioural approach'. In B. Stenfert Kroese, D. Dagnan and K. Loumidis (eds) *Cognitive Behavioural Therapy for People with Learning Disabilities.* London: Routledge.

Reed, J. (2003) 'Mental health care in prisons'. *British Journal of Psychiatry 182*, 287–8.

Reed, J. and Clements, J. (1989) 'Assessing the understanding of emotional states in a population of adolescents and young adults with mental handicaps'. *Journal of Mental Deficiency Research 33*, 229–233.

Rice, M.E., Harris, G.T., Quinsey, V.L. and Mireille, C. (1990) 'Planning treatment programs in secure psychiatric facilities'. *Law and Mental Health, International Perspectives 5*, 162–229. Oxford: Pergamon Press.

Rosenberg, S., Mueser, K., Jankowski, M. and Hamblen, J. (2002) 'Trauma exposure and PTSD in people with severe mental illness'. *PTSD Research Quarterly 13*, 3, Summer.

Rutherford, H. and Taylor, P. (in press) 'The transfer of female offenders with mental disorder from prison to hospital'. *Journal of Forensic Psychiatry and Psychology.*

Scott, S. (2000) 'The training needs of staff working with women in secure settings'. *Women in Secure Environments.* Conference Paper. Nottingham.

Scott, S. (2001) *The Politics and Experience of Ritual Abuse: Beyond Disbelief.* Buckingham: Open University Press.

Scott, S. and Parry-Crooke, G. (2001) 'Gender training needs of staff working in secure services'. *Mental Health Today*, October, 18–22.

Shaw, J., Appleby, L. and Baker, D. (2003) *Safer Prisons: A National Study of Prison Suicides by the National Confidential Inquiry into Suicides and Homicides by People with Mental Illness.* Manchester: University of Manchester.

Sinason. V. (1992) *Mental Handicap and the Human Condition: New Approaches from the Tavistock.* London: Free Association Books.

Singer, M. I., Bussey, J., Song, L. and Lunghofer, L. (1995) 'The psychosocial issues of women serving time in jail'. *Social Work 40*, 1, 103–113.

Singleton, N., Meltzer, H., Gatward, R., Coid, J. and Deasy, D. (1998) *Psychiatric Morbidity Among Prisoners in England and Wales.* London: HMSO.

Social Exclusion Unit (2002) *Reducing Re-offending by Ex-prisoners.* London: Social Exclusion Unit.

Stafford, P. (1999) *Defining Gender Issues: Redefining Women's Services*. London: WISH.

Storey, L. and Dale, C. (1999) *Nursing in Secure Environments*. London: UKCC.

Swanson, J.W., Holzer, C.E., Ganju, V.K. and Jonjo, R.T. (1990) 'Violence and psychiatric disorder in the community: evidence from the epidemiologic catchment area surveys'. *Hospital and Community Psychiatry 41*, 761–70.

Szivos, S. and Griffiths, E. (1992) 'Coming to terms with learning difficulties: the effects of groupwork and group processes on stigmatised identity'. In A. Waitman and S. Conboy-Hill (eds) *Psychotherapy and Mental Handicap*. London: Sage Publications.

Travers, R. (2003) 'Women patients in secure settings: (high) secure attachments'. *Royal College of Psychiatrists Annual Meeting (July)*. Presentation.

Turcan, M. (2001) 'Psychological interventions with women within a secure psychiatric service'. *XXVI International Congress on Law and Mental Health*. Abstract. Canada: Cheneliere/McGraw-Hill.

Van der Kolk, B., McFarlane, A.C. and Weisaeth, L. (1996) *Traumatic Stress: The Effects of Overwhelming Experience on Mind, Body and Society*. New York: Guilford Press.

Wahidin, A. (2000) 'Life behind the shadow: women's experience of prison in later life'. In R. Horn and S. Warner (eds) *Positive Directions for Women in Secure Environments*. Leicester: The British Psychological Society.

Waitman, A. and Conboy-Hill, S. (eds) (1992) *Psychotherapy and Mental Handicap*. London: Sage Publications.

Warner, S. (1996) 'Visibly special? Women, child sexual abuse and special hospitals'. In C. Hemingway (ed) *Special Women: The Experience of Women in the Special Hospital System*. London: Avebury Press.

Warner, S. (2000) 'The cost of containment'. *Forensic Update 62*, July, 5–9.

Watson, G., Scott, C. and Ragalsky, S. (1996) 'Refusing to be marginalized: groupwork in mental health services for women survivors of childhood sexual abuse'. *Journal of Community and Applied Social Psychology 6*, 5, 341–354.

Weiler, B.L. and Widom, C.S. (1996) 'Psychopathy and violent behaviour in abused and neglected young adults'. *Criminal Behaviour and Mental Health 6*, 253–227.

Widom, C. (1994) 'Does violence beget violence? A critical examination of the literature. Clarification of publishing history'. *Psychological Bulletin 115*, 287–295.

Widom, C. and Ames, M.A. (1994) 'Criminal consequences of childhood sexual victimisation'. *Child Abuse and Neglect 18*, 3030–318.

Williams, J. (1993) 'The importance of organising the therapeutic system'. *Clinical Psychology Forum*. March.

Williams, J. (1999) 'Social inequalities, mental health and mental health services'. In C. Newnes, G. Holmes and C. Dunn (eds) *This is Madness. A Critical Look at Psychiatry and the Future of Mental Health Services*. Ross-on-Wye: PCCS Books.

Williams, J., LeFrancois, B. and Copperman, J. (2001) *Mental Health Services that Work for Women: Survey Findings*. Canterbury: Tizard Centre, University of Kent.

Williams, J., Liebling, H., Lovelock, C., Chipchase, H. and Herbert, Y. (1998) 'Working with women in special hospitals'. *Feminism and Psychology 8*, 3, 357–369.

Williams, J. and Lindley, P. (1996) 'Working with mental health service users to change mental health services'. *Journal of Community and Applied Social Psychology 6*, 1, 1–14.

Williams, J., Scott, S. and Waterhouse, S. (2001) 'Mental health services for "difficult" women: reflections on some recent developments'. *Feminist Review 68*, Summer, 89–104.

Williams, J. and Waterhouse, S. (2000) *Women Whose Needs and Behaviours Challenge Mental Health Services in East Sussex: Findings and Recommendations.* Canterbury: Tizard Centre, University of Kent.

Williams, J. and Watson, G. (1991) 'Clinical psychology training in oppression?' *Feminism and Psychology 1*, 1, 55–101.

Williams, J. and Watson, G. (1997) 'Mental health services that empower women: the challenge to clinical psychology'. *Clinical Psychology Forum 100*, 11–18.

WISH (2000) *Good Girls: Surviving the Secure System.* London: WISH.

Worrall, A. (2000) 'Community sentences for women: where have they gone?' *Criminal Justice Matters 39*, Spring, 10–11.

Yorston, G. (1999) 'Aged and dangerous: old age forensic psychiatry'. *British Journal of Psychiatry 174*, 193–5.

Zlotkin, C. (1997) 'PTSD, PTSD comorbidity and childhood abuse among incarcerated women'. *Journal of Nervous and Mental Disease 185*, 761–763.

List of Contributors

Nikki Jeffcote is a clinical psychologist working in the medium secure service of West London Mental Health NHS Trust. She has had a specialist interest in the care and treatment needs of women in forensic settings since carrying out research (published under her previous surname, Gorsuch) on the healthcare wing of HMP Holloway. She has been involved in the development of NHS medium secure services for women since 1998 and works with both women and men in hospital and community settings.

Tessa Watson is a music therapist and lecturer. She trained as a music therapist in 1989 at Roehampton, and since qualifying has worked extensively in adult mental health and learning disability services. Her current clinical work is in a community team for people with learning disabilities. Tessa also works at University of Surrey Roehampton where she is Course Convenor for Music Therapy postgraduate programmes.

Gwen Adshead is a forensic psychiatrist and psychotherapist working at Broadmoor Hospital. After her forensic training, she lectured in Victimology at the Institute of Psychiatry, carrying out research into post-traumatic stress disorder, before training as a group analyst and psychotherapist. She is currently involved in a research project into the attachment characteristics of maltreating mothers. Gwen's other main interest is ethical dilemmas in forensic psychiatry.

Anne Aiyegbusi is Nurse Consultant for Women's Services at Broadmoor Hospital, West London Mental Health NHS Trust. She has worked in high and medium security mental health services for over 20 years, in a range of nursing roles. Her particular interests are forensic psychotherapy, attachment theory, psychological trauma and the emotional impact on nursing staff of work with traumatised women offenders.

Miranda Barber works as a forensic clinical psychologist at Awen Women's Service, Llanarth Court Hospital, an independent provider of medium secure care for mentally disordered offenders. She has an interest in the general area of trauma, and in the clinical application of attachment theory to mental health.

Amanda Bragg is a senior occupational therapist in the women's secure service at West London Mental Health Trust. She has seven years' experience in both community mental health and hospital-based rehabilitation in Australia and the UK. Her clinical interests include women's mental health, cross-cultural practice and community resettlement.

Carole Bressington is a Broadmoor survivor and former WISH worker. She previously worked for the NHS in a variety of nursing posts for almost 20 years. An accredited associate trainer, she delivers Inequality Agenda's gender awareness training to multi-disciplinary teams. Carole lives, and occasionally writes, in Somerset.

Sarah Devereux is an occupational therapist who previously worked in community arts. Since qualifying she has worked for West London Mental Health Trust, in the Forensic Division, and for the past two years for the women's service. She has recently returned from sabbatical in Mexico and India.

Tim Lambert is a consultant forensic psychiatrist and general adult psychiatrist at West London Mental Health NHS Trust. He is honorary clinical lecturer at Imperial College of Science, Technology and Medicine, and Clinical Director of the Local Secure and Specialist Rehabilitation Directorate, which encompasses a secure women's ward.

Tony Maden is Professor of Forensic Psychiatry at Imperial College, London and Clinical Director of Services for Dangerous and Severe Personality Disorder at West London Mental Health Trust. He has worked on surveys of women in prison and in secure hospitals. One of his main interests is the application of standardised risk assessment in clinical practice. He likes to think that his attitude to risk assessment is enthusiastic but not gung ho.

Anna Motz is a consultant clinical psychologist for Oxfordshire Mental Healthcare NHS Trust and currently works in a low secure unit. She is the Secretary of the International Association of Forensic Psychotherapy. She has a particular interest in the assessment and treatment of female offenders and women who self-harm. Her book, *The Psychology of Female Violence: Crimes Against the Body*, was published in 2001.

Laila Namdarkhan is a regional manager, consultant and trainer with Women in Secure Hospitals (WISH). She was previously a senior manager and lead nurse for a large NHS Trust. Laila has an MA in Gender and Society, and is a board member of YWCA and Women's Link. She is a national trainer for Inequality Agenda's gender awareness training.

Les Petrie trained as a registered mental health nurse in Scotland. He has worked in psychiatric intensive care and forensic services in London, including a women's secure service. Les is currently Team Leader for a Women's Forensic Service at Fromeside Clinic, Bristol, where he is developing a dedicated women's service. Les has a BSc in Nursing, a Post Graduate Diploma in Management studies and has also trained in Dialectic Behavioural Therapy. He is currently working towards an MSc in Pschoanalytic studies. Les has a keen interest in developing a training approach for supporting staff working with women patients.

Carole Rowley is a nurse manager currently managing forensic services for women with learning disabilities at Brooklands, North Warwickshire Primary Care Trust. She is presently working towards an MSc in Psychodynamic Counselling.

Helen Rutherford is a consultant forensic psychiatrist at West London Mental Health NHS Trust. She has considerable experience of working with both male and female patients in high secure hospitals. She has had a specialist interest in the needs of female mentally disordered offenders since working on the Healthcare Unit of HMP Holloway in the 1990s.

Sara Scott is a principal research officer with Barnardo's. After ten years in social action broadcasting she obtained a PhD in Sociology in the mid-1990s. Her main research interests concern gender, violence and mental health. She was previously Director (1999–2001) of the Gender Training Initiative at the University of Liverpool. Her book, *The Politics and Experience of Ritual Abuse: Beyond Disbelief,* was published in 2001.

Jackie Short is a consultant forensic and general adult psychiatrist and a trained general and psychiatric nurse. She is the clinical lead for Awen Women's Service, a secure service for women in the independent sector, developed in collaboration with NHS commissioners and clinicians. She works on a number of committees for women's mental health issues.

Su Thrift, clinical psychologist, has worked in learning disability services since gaining her Clinical Doctorate in 1996. She is the psychological lead in forensic services for men and women with learning disability at Brooklands, North Warwickshire Primary Care Trust. Her professional interests include sexual trauma and its sequelae, loss, violence to others and the self, and psychodynamic psychotherapy.

Ray Travers is a consultant forensic psychiatrist and Clinical Director of the National High Secure Women's Directorate at Rampton Hospital. He qualified as a doctor in 1984, and as a psychiatrist in 1991, and worked as a consultant forensic psychiatrist at Ashworth Hospital before taking up his position at Rampton in 1998. His special interest is the provision of services for women with severe personality disorder.

Maja Turcan is a consultant forensic clinical psychologist at West London Mental Health NHS Trust. She works at Three Bridges Medium Secure Unit and the Forensic Psychology Outpatient service. She has particular responsibility for the provision of psychological services to women patients.

Jennie Williams is a clinical psychologist and Director of Inequality Agenda, a specialist organisation that supports mental health providers in responding progressively to the mental health needs of women. She contributes through Department of Health committees to the implementation of the National Women's Mental Health Strategy and to putting equality issues on the agenda of workforce planning.

Subject Index

Author Index

3 5282 00586 0781